William George Black

Folk-Medicine

a Chapter in the History Of Culture

William George Black

Folk-Medicine
a Chapter in the History Of Culture

ISBN/EAN: 9783744768658

Printed in Europe, USA, Canada, Australia, Japan

Cover: Foto ©ninafisch / pixelio.de

More available books at **www.hansebooks.com**

The Folk-Lore Society,

FOR COLLECTING AND PRINTING

RELICS OF POPULAR ANTIQUITIES, &c.

ESTABLISHED IN

THE YEAR MDCCCLXXVIII.

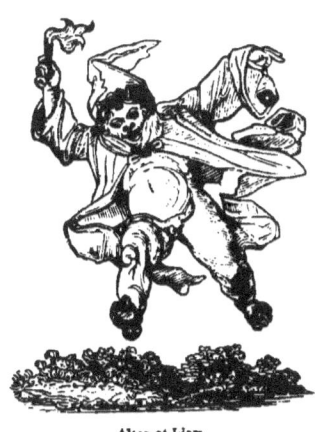

Alter et Idem.

PUBLICATIONS
OF
THE FOLK-LORE SOCIETY.

XII.

FOLK-MEDICINE;

A CHAPTER IN

THE HISTORY OF CULTURE.

BY

WILLIAM GEORGE BLACK,
F.S.A.Scot.

LONDON:
PUBLISHED FOR THE FOLK-LORE SOCIETY BY
ELLIOT STOCK, 62, PATERNOSTER ROW, E.C.

1883.

To the Memory of

C. B. B.

THIS BOOK IS DEDICATED

BY

HER SON.

CONTENTS.

CHAP.
I. INTRODUCTION: ORIGIN OF DISEASE . 1
II. TRANSFERENCE OF DISEASE , . 31
III. SYMPATHY AND ASSOCIATION OF IDEAS . . 49
IV. NEW BIRTH AND SACRIFICE . . . 65
V. OUR LORD AND THE SAINTS IN FOLK-MEDICINE . . 75
VI. CHARMS CONNECTED WITH DEATH OR THE GRAVE . 95
VII. COLOUR 108
VIII. (1) NUMBER—(2) INFLUENCE OF THE SUN AND MOON . 118
IX. PERSONAL CURES 136
X. ANIMAL CURES 148
XI. SPECIFIC CHARMS: (1) MAGIC WRITINGS—(2) RINGS . . 165
XII. DOMESTIC FOLK-MEDICINE 178
XIII. THE PLACE OF FOLK-MEDICINE IN THE STUDY OF CIVILIZATION 204

PREFACE.

"FOLK-MEDICINE" comprehends charms, incantations, and traditional habits and customs relative to the preservation of health and the cure of disease, practised now or formerly at home and abroad; an attempt has been made in the following pages also to classify the explanations of the cause of disease which come to light in folk-lore. I would refer to Chapter XIII. for my reasons for differing from certain conclusions to which Mr. Herbert Spencer has given the weight of his authority on subjects intimately associated with several classes of Folk-Medicine.

Through the courtesy of many correspondents, known and unknown, I have been enabled to make use of notes which in several instances have not before appeared in print. I have endeavoured in every case to indicate my authority for the folk-lore embodied in my text, and should I in any case have failed to do so I must ask my readers to believe that there has been no intentional neglect. A list is appended of the chief works consulted. When the MS. left my hands no part of Grimm's great work, *Deutsche Mythologie*, had been translated, otherwise I should, of course, have availed myself of English words. As it is, I have added in most cases a second reference to the translation by Mr. Stallybrass, when a quotation has been made from the *first* volume; the second volume of Mr. Stallybrass's translation has been too recently issued to allow of my making use of it in the same way. M. Lenormant's *La Magie chez les Chaldéens* has also been translated since I first referred to its pages. The publications of the Folk-Lore Society have been of great service, and also the works of Dr. Tylor and Sir John Lubbock.

Special acknowledgment for notes, books, references, and counsel, must be made to Dr. Tylor, Mr. A. Lang, Professor Veitch, and Professor Young, of Glasgow University; Professor Lindsay, of the Free Church College, Glasgow; Miss Guernsey, Rochester, U.S.A.; Mr. W. H. Patterson, Belfast; and the Rev. G. S. Streitfeild, Louth.

Mr. Gomme and Mr. Robert Guy, Glasgow, have read all the proof sheets and revises, and have favoured me with many suggestions. To Mr. Gomme I am, in common with all the other members of the Folk-Lore Society, under great obligations for unfailing courtesy; but I trust he will allow me to bear special testimony to his untiring desire to promote the best interests of the study of Folk-Lore. The fault of any errors or mis-statements must entirely rest upon myself; that there are such I cannot but believe; that there were not more is due to the careful and valued criticism of Mr. Gomme and Mr. Guy.

WILLIAM GEORGE BLACK.

1, Alfred Terrace, Glasgow.
7th May, 1883.

FOLK-MEDICINE.

CHAPTER I.

INTRODUCTION.

N approaching a subject involved in great obscurity the first duty of a writer must be to strike a note of warning. This is specially necessary when the primitive conceptions of the origin of disease, as suggested or evinced by existing folk-lore and kindred conceptions in Folk-Medicine generally, are to be considered. However well authenticated the facts may seem to be, any conjecture founded on them should, in the present state of our knowledge, be tendered with caution, and only accepted after careful consideration, for generalization on the subject of superstitions must be always perilous.

But, while this is so, it must be obvious that no progress can be made at all unless we grapple with such facts as we have. We have some data to go upon. The possibility of arriving at definite rules in other branches has been proved, over and over again, by the students at home and on the Continent, who have presented the world with studies at once exact and liberal—exact, because they are the fruit of untiring zeal in seeking authentic sources of information; liberal, because the bare facts have been collectively illuminated by a light which could have had no existence had generalization not been attempted.

It cannot be altogether vain to hope that reasons for investigation, of a precise kind, may also be found in the beliefs which are treated of in the following pages, and, although it has always been with hesitation that I have allowed myself to do more than place my notes before my readers, yet these beliefs, like living things, have a beginning and a reason, and some indulgence may perhaps be allowed to one who finds his barque sailing among strange islands.

I may go further, and affirm that in the matter of that which follows there is much which deserves attention. The facts are, indeed, so scattered up and down the pages of travels and histories, of voyages and tales, that it is easy to excuse even a man interested in the proper study of mankind having but hazy notions of the thoughts of his rural countrymen on such a subject; yet, apart from other things, we have in the Folk-Medicine which still exists the unwritten record of the beginning of the practice of medicine and surgery.

Medical science, like everything else, like our language and our mental conceptions, is the reward of long seeking after light. It has been built up from generation to generation by one people after another, by one man finding out the errors of a predecessor, and a third improving upon both. The tendency of all such developments, however, is to follow the conqueror's plan, and burn the ships. In nature the branch bursts from the tree, and the leaf bursts from the branch, but the growth of the branch does not make the tree less useful, nor does the leaf detract from the branch's merit. In the processes of men's minds, on the other hand, things go differently. When a thought has borne a new fruit, a new thought,—the new thought succeeds to the place of the old, as one king succeeds another on a throne. The old idea is consigned at once to the limbo of the forgotten. It seems useless, unnecessary, cumbering, dead, beside the new. In course of time, therefore, a work of no small difficulty lies before the student or philosopher who attempts to trace the growth of a single science if written records are wanting. It has not been my intention to illustrate of purpose, by Folk-Medicine, the development of medical science; this is not the place for, nor am I competent to undertake, such investigation, but I do not hesitate to say that the early history of medical science, as of all other developments of culture, can be studied more narrowly and more accurately in the folk-lore of this and other countries than some students of modern science and exact modern records may think possible. Mr. Spencer has said * the course of social change is so irregular, involved, and rhythmical, that it cannot be judged of in its general direction by inspecting any small portion of it; but, while this is admitted, when we consider an earlier remark of the same writer,† that true appreciation of the successive facts which an individual life, even, presents is generally hindered by inability to grasp the gradual processes by which ultimate effects are produced, it becomes clear that to elucidate the contending and conflicting facts, as well as may be, by the aid of comparative folk-lore, is at least one reason why such works as deal with the history of culture may advantageously be compiled and consulted.

After the first shock of death the natural task of man was to seek a reason for the sudden lack of life in one who, but a short time before, had gone about the world as did his brothers still. It must soon have been suggested that the rude weapon of the chase which had missed its aim had some volition of its own, or that some mysterious influence, which had protected the victim from injury before, had been absent or unfriendly. Such a thing as natural death was probably for a long time inconceivable, as it appears still inconceivable to such peoples as the Prairie Indians, who treat all diseases alike, since they must all alike have been caused by one evil spirit. In the South

* *The Study of Sociology*, 7th edition, p. 105.
† *Ibid.* p. 102.

Pacific no one is supposed to die a natural death unless decrepit with extreme old age, and in South Africa, according to Chapman, and Philip, and Cameron, it is thought that no man dies from natural causes, or by Heaven's decree; he must have been either poisoned or bewitched.* Instances might be gathered from all quarters of the world where man in some measure retains the primitive thought, and traces of the belief may be found in modern folk-lore, perhaps also in the anxiety which is shown to account for any manner of illness by some external cause.

Many are the reasons, as D'Iharace says, that have tended to errors in medicine, "teles que les préjugés de l'éducation, la disposition naturelle à l'erreur, les fausses idées, la crédulité, la prévention pour l'antiquité, l'autorité, l'exemple, et plusieurs autres, que les dialectriciens connoissent," † but it is not necessary here to do more than refer to the three great sources of disease and death which have commended themselves to peoples in search of some other explanation of the suspension of life than is offered by belief in natural death. These are—

(1.) The anger of an offended external spirit;
(2.) The supernatural powers of a human enemy;
(3.) The displeasure of the dead.

(1.) Nothing can be more easily aroused than the anger of a spirit. In L'ien-chow, in the province of Kwang-si, if a man hits his foot against a stone, and afterwards falls sick, his family know that there was a demon in the stone, and they immediately repair to the place where it lies with offerings of fruit, wine, rice, and incense, and worship. After this the

---

* Lubbock, *Origin of Civilization*, p. 29; Gill, *Myths and Songs from the South Pacific*, p. 35; Chapman, *Travels in Africa*, vol. i. p. 47; Philip, *South Africa*, vol. i. p. 118; Cameron, *Across Africa*, vol. i. p. 116; *Christian Express* (Lovedale, S. Africa,) October, 1878, p. 11.

† D'Iharace, *Erreurs populaires sur la Médecine*, 1783, p. iii.

patient recovers.* The aborigines of Australia ascribe small-pox to a spirit who delights in mischief; in Cambodia all disease is attributed to an evil spirit who torments the sick man. Among the Dayacks of Borneo to have been smitten by a spirit is to be ill; " sickness may be caused by invisible spirits inflicting invisible wounds with invisible spears, or entering men's bodies and driving them raving mad." " As in normal conditions the man's soul, inhabiting his body, is held to give it life, to think, speak, and act through it, so an adaptation of the self-same principle explains abnormal conditions of body or mind, by considering the new symptoms as due to the operation of a second soul-like being, a strange spirit. The possessed man, tossed and shaken in fever, pained and wrenched as though some live creature were tearing or twisting him within, rationally finds a personal spiritual cause for his sufferings," and a name for the possessing demon, " which it can declare when it speaks in its own voice and character through his organs of speech," so implicit is the sick man's belief in the personality.† The disease spirit having been thus created, we are not surprised that the native Australians regard their demon Biam as black and deformed, since he is the inflictor of small-pox, although neither Wuotan in Scandinavian mythology, nor Apollo in classic, share his repulsiveness, and yet from both, as Grimm points out, came severe illnesses and pestilence as well as cures.‡ Personification of disease is general. In Ceylon the great demon of disease is associated with a peculiar legend. His father was a king who, believing his queen to have been faithless to him,

---

* Dennys, *Folk-Lore of China*, p. 96. Cf. "Even Siva is worshipped as a stone, especially that Siva who will afflict a child with epileptic fits, and then, speaking by its voice, will announce that he is Panchânana, the Five-faced, and is punishing the child for insulting his image."—Tylor, *Primitive Culture*, vol. ii. p. 150.

† Tylor, *Primitive Culture*, vol. ii. pp. 113, 114, 116.

‡ Conway, *Demonology and Devil-Lore*, vol. i. p. 98 ; Grimm, *Deutsche Mythologie*, vol. i. p. 123 ; Stallybrass, vol. i. p. 149.

ordered her to be cut in two, one part of her body to be thrown to the dogs, and one part hung upon a tree. The queen before this sentence was executed is reported to have said, "If this charge be false, may the child in my womb be born this instant a demon, and may that demon destroy the whole of this city and its unjust king." Nevertheless the sentence was executed. But a wonder happened. The severed parts reunited, and a child was born, who repaired to the burying-place of the city and there fattened on the corpses. "Then he proceeded to inflict mortal diseases upon the city, and had nearly depopulated it, when the gods Iswara and Sekkra interfered, descending to subdue him in the disguise of mendicants." He had eighteen principal attendants, the first of whom was the Demon of Madness.* This seems to have been almost as dreadful a monster as that which appeared in a dream to a Chinese emperor who flourished about 700 A.D. One day when he was ill, he dreamt he saw a blue half-naked devil coming into his palace. He stole the empress's perfume bag, and also the emperor's flute, which was made of precious stones, and flew off with them to the palace roof. Suddenly there appeared another blue devil, but of giant stature, having a black leather high boot on one foot, the other being bare. He had on a blue gown. One arm was bare, and wielded a massive sword. His head was like that of a bull. This fierce-looking monster seized the little one, and with a blow made an end of him. The emperor was greatly flattered at being visited by such a distinguished, although unearthly, personage, and waking up *found his disease gone.* He called a painter to paint for him what he had seen in his dream, and it was executed so faithfully that the emperor ordered two hundred ounces of gold to be given him, and that copies of the painting should be distributed through the whole empire, so that all the people might know and pay due respect

---

* Conway, *Demonology*, vol. i. pp. 261, 262.

to this blue bull-headed demon. To this day he holds a conspicuous place in the temples of the people.*

As the disease spirits of less cultured men than Chinese emperors would be proportionally more horrible, we can believe it is with gratification the Orang Laut, like the Khonds of Orissa, contemplate the barricades of thorns and bushes, and ditches and stinking oil with which they endeavour to keep off the goddess of small pox. So too among the Betschvaria, that disease may be averted, or prevented from entering their town, if a painted stone be planted in the ground in the middle of the entrance to the town (each town being inclosed by a hedge of bushes), or if a crossbar, duly smeared with medicine, be put up at the entrance. "When this is done, they imagine themselves safe." In the same sense we read in the *Medicina de Quadrupedibus* of Sextus Placitus, when he refers to the virtues of the neat, "take his liver, divide it, and delve it down at the turnings round of thy land boundaries, and of thy borough wall foundations, and hide the heart at thy borough gates; then thou and thine shall be released in health to go about and home to return; all pestilence shall be driven away, and what was ere done shall naught scathe, and there shall little mischief from fire." †

This personification of disease, this theory that "jeder todesengel ist der Tod selbst, der seine leute abholt " is illustrated in the imaginative conception of the same dread power, which we find in times more ancient than those of Sextus Placitus, " To the mind of the Israelite," says Mr. Tylor, " death and pestilence took the personal form of the destroying angel who smote the doomed."‡ And in Justinian's time men saw brazen barques with black and headless men on board, and, where the vessel touched, there the pestilence appeared.

* Dennys, *Folk-Lore of China*, p. 84.
† Tylor, *Primitive Culture*, vol. ii. pp. 115, 116; South African *Folk-Lore Journal*, vol. i. p. 34; Cockayne, *Leechdoms*, vol. i. pp. 329-331.
‡ Grimm, *Deutsche Mythologie*, vol. ii. p. 989, *et seq.*; Tylor, *Primitive Culture*, vol. i. p. 267; 2 Samuel xxiv. 16; 2 Kings xix. 35.

Naturally when the fear of this personified disease overcame man he strove to make friends with his enemy by giving flattering names, "so heisst es das gute, das gesegnete, das selige oder die seuche wird gevatterin angeredet,"—as among the Greeks the furies were called Eumenides, and among ourselves the fairies—the mediaeval descendants of the jinns and demons of the East and the giants and monsters of the South—were so long styled "the good people," as in course of time to acquire all the good attributes which should pertain to such a name. It was beyond the imaginative power of man in any country, however, to cast this rosy light over the grim death angel himself. He was called the Good and the Blessed, but it was impossible to associate with the grim reality—except in the language of hyperbolical poetry—the magic human meaning of the words. We have, therefore, and in modern literature, a twofold personification of death, which it is difficult to distinguish although not impossible to comprehend. Like the good people, the lineal descendants of a superhuman race, we have death the reaper and death the brother of sleep, but we have also the grim skeleton; we have, in a word, in our mind, at once both the terror-striking "Pest" and the mysterious "Good." And this double conception we owe to a time so ancient that our brains almost reel at the thought of the thousand minds required to give rounded significance to an idea.

The Assyrians and Babylonians believed that the world was swarming with noxious spirits, who, in food or drink, might be swallowed, and so cause disease. Three hundred were of heaven, and six hundred of earth. Exorcisms were employed to expel the spirits, apparently in all cases, for no mention has been found of medicine. "The baneful charm,"—runs one of these exorcisms—"like an evil demon, acts against the man. The voice that defiles acts upon him. The maleficent voice acts upon him. The baneful charm is a spell that originates sickness." These exorcisms appear to have been borrowed by the Assyrians from the primitive population of Babylonia.* Among the Finns, whose language resembles the agglutinative language of the early Babylonians, all disease is regarded as the work of a demon, and the tietjat (savants) and noijat are said to have the power of chasing from the body diseases, "considérées comme des êtres personnels, par le moyen de leurs formules, de leurs chants, et aussi de breuvages enchantés dans la composition desquels ils faisaient entrer des substances réellement pharmaceutiques; ils étaient les seuls médecins de la nation."†

"Les Kirghises," says M. Lenormant, whose citations and remarks on this point are particularly interesting, "s'addressent de même à leurs sorciers ou *baksy*, pour chasser les démons et guérir ainsi les maladies qu'on suppose produites par eux. Pour cela, ils fouettent le malade jusqu'au sang et lui crachent au visage. Toute affection est à leurs yeux un être personnel. Cette idée est pareillement si accréditée chez les Tchouvaches, qu'ils assurent que le moindre oubli des devoirs est puni par une maladie que leur envoie Tchémen, démon dont le nom est une forme altérée de Schaïtan. On retrouve à peu près la même opinion chez les Tchouktchis ; ces sauvages ont recours, pour délivrer les malades, aux plus bizarres conjurations."‡ Grimm quotes from a Finnish song,— "einen alten frau, neun knaben geboren werden ; werwolf, schlange, risi (?) eidechse, nachtmar, gliedschmerz, gichtschmerz, milzstechen, bauchgrimmen. Diese krankheiten sind also geschwister venderblicher umgehauer ; in dem lied wird dann die letze derselben hervorgehoben und beschworen."§ That a person was bewitched, however, sometimes needed proof, but Cotta, in his *Tryal of Witchcraft*,

---

* *Records of the Past*, vol. i. p. 131 ; vol. iii. pp. 139, 147.

† Lenormant, *La Magié chez les Chaldéens*, p. 219 (quoting Lönnrot, *Abhandlung über die magische Medicin der Finnen*).

‡ Lenormant, *Ibid.* p. 188 (*Levchine, Description des hordes et des steppes des Kirghiz-Kazaks*, pp. 356, 358 ; *Nouvelles Annales des Voyages*, 5° série, t. iv. p. 191).

§ Grimm, *Deutsche Mythologie*, vol. ii. p. 972 ; Lenormant, *Ibid.* pp. 232, 233.

made clear the two ways by which, as he says, reason may detect if the sick have been bewitched. The first way is by such things as are subject and manifest to the learned physician only; the second is by such things as are subject and manifest to the vulgar view; that is to say—first, by the preternatural appearance of the disease; and secondly, the inefficacy of the remedies.* Hodgson records a more elaborate mode of discovery practised among the Bodo and Dhimal. The exorcist sets thirteen loaves round the patient; these represent the gods, one of whom must have been offended. The exorcist then holds a pendulum attached to his thumb by a string, until the god, much besought, declares himself by making the pendulum swing towards his representative loaf. The chief of Queensland demons makes himself visible at great assemblies, and, as he is not only the author of disease, but also of mischief and wisdom, he fitly makes his appearance as a serpent. To the present day there are people in Great Britain who have seen the disease serpent when exhibiting himself in the annoying illness called *shingles*. One physician suffered so extremely as in moments of excessive pain to touch the rough scales of the imagined serpent with his hand.†

It is more natural to regard the spirits as each appointed to a special charge, as do the Mintira of the Malay peninsula (whose most feared demons are tree-demons), than as causing all diseases impartially because they simply happened to be diseases. Dr. William Ramsay, a court physician of the seventeenth century, thought that magicians and witches, as "the imps and instruments of Satan," might be instrumental in causing worms especially‡. One wonders if this repute has any connection with the Polish naming of the *wiese leute* Würmer, those who "in den menschen krankheiten verursachen." The connection

* Cited by Spalding, *Elizabethan Demonology*, p. 64.

† Hodgson, *Abor. of India*, p. 170, cited by Tylor, *Primitive Culture*, vol. i. pp. 114, 115, 378, 278-9.

‡ Tylor, *Primitive Culture*, vol. ii. pp. 115, 196; Ramsay's Ελμινθολογια, p. 79 (1668). Ramsay supports his theory with many quaint tales, citing Boisardus, *De Divinatione*, &c.

INTRODUCTION. 11

would certainly be strengthened by the fact that, while some peoples have taught that toothache is the work of a devil (perhaps of a particular devil, and as the New Zealanders gave a separate deity to each part of the body, Tonga, to cause headache and sickness, Moko-Tiki, pains in the chest, and so on, the Christians allotted saints and devils*), others have declared it to be the work of a worm; but to this we shall refer later on. The Assyrians shared the same apportioning belief as the New Zealanders, it appears, for among their demons, to which reference has above been made, some injured the head, some the hands and feet.† The Zulus, while believing in spirits, lay special stress on the killing propensities of the rainbow. "When it devours a person, he dies a sudden or violent death. All persons that die badly, by falls, by drowning, or by wild beasts, die because the rainbow has devoured their ka-la or spirit. On devouring persons it becomes thirsty, and comes down to drink, when it is seen in the sky drinking water. Therefore, when people see the rainbow they say, 'The rainbow has come to drink water. Look out, some one or other will die violently by an evil death.'" This is the belief of the Karens of Birma, and the Zulus similarly say, "The rainbow is disease. If it rests on a man something will happen to him."‡ Well might these peoples wish the rainbow were as accommodating as the demon in China, who may be pacified by a meal, after it has entered the body of a relative of the sick man, and has reproved him for the sin which

* Biesters, cited by Grimm, *Deutsche Mythologie*, vol. ii. p. 968. Taylor, *New Zealand and its Inhabitants*, p. 34. Lubbock, *Origin of Civilization*, p. 30.
† *Records of the Past*, vol. iii. p. 140.
‡ Mason, *Karens*, in *Jour. As. Soc.* Bengal, 1865, part ii. p. 217; Callaway, *Zulu Tales*, vol. i. p. 294; Tylor, *Primitive Culture*, vol. i. p. 266. Lightning, it might be expected, would be universally regarded as a terrible demon, but "einen blitzerschlagnen preisen die Osseten glücklich und glauben, Elias (Ilia) habe ihn zu sich genommen; die hinterbliebenen erheben freudengeschrei, singen und tanzen um den leichnam, alles strömt herzu, schliesst sich dem reihen an und singt: 'O Ellai, Ellai eldaer tschoppoi' (O Elias, Elias, herr der felsengipfel)."—Grimm, *Deutsche Mythologie*, vol. i. p. 145. *Stallybrass*, vol. i. p. 174.

had brought the disease upon him.* To get actual knowledge of the visit of the spirits, "wenn einen kranken die weissen leute quälen wird in Polen freitags ein lager von erbsenstroh gemacht, laken gespreitet und der kranke darauf gelegt. Dann trägt einer ein sieb mit asche auf dem rücken, geht um den kranken herum, und lässt die asche auslaufen, so dass das ganze lager davon umstreut wird. Frühmorgens *zählt man alle striche auf der asche*, und stillschweigends, ohne unterwegs zu grüssen, hintenbringt sie einer der klugen frau, die nun mittel verschreibt," and "in der asche drücken sich die spuren der geiste ab, wie man auch den erdmännlein asche streut."†

Some tribes of Indians have tried to appease the anger of offended water-spirits by offerings of such things as they themselves most prized. A mysterious virtue attached to water-lilies among the Frisians, and Dutch boys are said to be extremely careful in plucking or handling them, for, if a boy fall with the flowers in his possession, he immediately becomes subject to fits.‡

Paralysis was explained in Shetland, in former days, by saying that an evil spirit had touched the limb, or that the sound limb had been abstracted and an insensible mass substituted,§ with the same reasoning as had Africans when they spoke of certain aged persons as having taken and eaten the spirits of five individuals.

It is a natural and well-known fact that the gods of one nation become the devils of their conquerors or successors. The Northern deities were only partially saved by the recognition of a Christ in Baldur, as the Roman deities by the identification of

---

* *Strange Stories from a Chinese Studio*, vol. ii. p. 131.

† Grimm, *Deutsche Mythologie*, vol. ii. p. 975. For another use of ashes "wenn man erkennen soll dass einer bezaubert sey," see *Joh. Agricola in Chirurg.* par. v. p. 571, quoted in Martius, *De Magica Naturali*, p. 40.

‡ Franklin, *Journey to the Polar Sea*, vol. ii. p. 245; Tylor, *Primitive Culture*, vol. ii. p. 192; *Notes and Queries*, 1st S. vol. iii. p. 387; *Choice Notes (Folk-Lore)*, p. 7.

§ Dalyell, *Darker Superstitions of Scotland*, p. 304; Hibbert, *Shetland Islands*, p. 431.

the Virgin Mary with the highest virtues of the ancient queens of Heaven. "La plus grande partie de la magie du moyen âge," says Lenormant, "a ce caractère et perpétue les rites populaires et superstitieux du paganisme, à l'état d'opérations mystérieuses et diaboliques de sorcellerie." This is seen all over the world, as in Ceylon since the conversion of the island to Buddhism, "les anciens dieux du civaïsme sont devenus des démons et leur culte des sortilèges coupables que pratiquent les seuls enchanteurs."* We may conclude that in England the devil has long represented much of old paganism still existing. He seems to have been regarded almost as the head of the medical profession; "the devil," Sir George Mackenzie said only two hundred years ago, "may inflict diseases, which is an effect he may occasion applicando activa passivis [by applying actives to passives] and by the same means he may likewise cure . . . . and not only may he cure diseases laid on by himself, as Wierus observes, but even natural diseases, since he knows the natural causes and the origin of even those natural diseases better than physicians can, who are not present when diseases are contracted, and who, *being younger than he*, must have less experience. And it is as untrue that Pirius Thomas observes, who asserts that cures performed by the devil cannot continue, since his cures are not natural."

Conrad under head § xix. "magia effectorea est admirandorum operum realium, auxilio Diaboli productio," discriminates as follows:—

"Est autem illa ipsa, respectu subjectorum circa quæ occupata est, partim *utilis*, partim *inutilis* s. *noxia*, quamvis utraque ad hominum tam temporalem quam æternam tendat perniciem. Ad priorem classem spectat curatio vulnerum, morborum, abactio Spectrorum (wenn ein Teufel den andern austreibet) aliorumque malorum averruncatio. Ad posteriorem, tempesta-

---

* Lenormant, *La Magie chez les Chaldéens*, pp. 69-70.

tum horrendarum ventorumque tumultuantium excitatio, frugum perditio, hominum pecorumque læsio, &c." *

A Scotch witch, who was famous for her cures of sick children, used to say as she administered the remedy, "I give thee it in Godis name, but the devil give thee good of it."

(2.) Next in importance to the theory of the origin of disease referred to above, if with propriety we may place one above another, or assign a greater or less importance, was the theory which attributed all diseases or bodily misfortune to the supernatural powers of a human enemy. It is the general alternative among races in a low state of civilization, and to the present day South American Indians, Kols of Nagpore, and Kaffirs of Koussa, speak with dread of the powers of the sorcerer, of the charmers who can bring evil or good upon a man.† Even in this century newspaper readers must be aware that wise women whose curses are feared, and whose advice is craved, are not uncommon in England. I know of a professional charmer for toothache having practised in Cheshire within the last twenty years; in Lancashire consumptive patients and paralytics are often said to be bewitched; and Mr. Gregor, writing of the early part of this century, speaks of a class of people whose curses or *prayers*, as they were called, were much dreaded. To incur the displeasure of one of these people was to call down his prayers, and those prayers were speedily followed by bodily disease or accident, or by disaster to property, or by the miscarrying of some undertaking—by misfortune of some kind or other. "The remark was quite common, 'So-and-so got his leg broken aifter So-and-so curst 'im.' 'So-and-so never hid a weels day aifter he fell oot wi' So-and-so.' 'Ill health's never been out o' So-and-so's hoose sin he keest oot wee So-and-so.' 'The beggar-wife's

---

* Elias Conrad, *Disputatio Physica exhibens;* i. *Doctrinam de Magia*, ii. *Thearemata Miscellanea*, 1661. See Ramsay, Ελμινθολογια, pp. 54 *et seq.*

† Lichtenstein, *Travels in S. Africa*, vol. ii. p. 255; Stevenson, *Travels in S. America*, vol. i. p. 60; Lubbock, *Origin of Civilization*, pp. 32, 224, 371.

malison hiz lichtit on So-and-so's hoose for pittin' hir in 'ir bairn oot in a nicht o' blin' drift.'"* If "dark working sorcerers that change the mind, soul-killing witches that deform the body," were thus fearfully regarded within our own days, it is not wonderful that in other countries and in earlier times the trade of disease-making, or invoking, was a decidedly favourite one. The governing class was at once medical, legal, and religious; the chief, the priest, and the medicine man were one. Disease being primarily attributed to an external supernatural power, who might, as Lenormant says of the god of the Finns, not only be the god of waters and air, but also "l'esprit d'où découle toute vie, le maître des enchantements favorables, l'adversaire et le vainqueur de toutes les personnifications du mal, le souverain possesseur de toute science," † it is the duty of the priests to watch over the actions of this deity, yet the chief function of their body as a profession is, we find, to discriminate in matters of medicine. A priest, if he cannot or does not see fit to trace the disease to a direct imposition on the part of an external spirit, should be able to point out a person who has occasioned the mischief, and if a spite be cherished against any one his fate is practically sealed. The office of magician is even in some places hereditary; the son succeeds the father, if the father has managed to save himself, but if it is suspected that a wizard has practised against the welfare of a chief (though in many cases the chief is himself the head priest and doctor in one) the short and speedy way in Central Africa for preventing a repetition of the attempt is to destroy his whole household with the head offender. Often when suffering agonies these magicians boast of their exploits, and die with vaunts of the deaths they have caused, and the rainfalls they have prevented. The Australians track their sorcerers by watching an insect which is said

---

* *Lancashire Folk-lore*, p. 164; *Journal* Anthropological Institute, vol. iii. p. 267. See also Gregor's *Folk-Lore of North-East of Scotland*, p. 35.

† Lenormant, *La Magie chez les Chaldéens*, p. 222.

to crawl from the grave of a bewitched man in the direction of the house of the wizard who caused his death, and other peoples have their modes of discovery.*

But curses and denunciation are not the only means by which nations of thought have found their magicians work their evil will. There are more elaborate ways, and more effectual, in so far as they appeal to secret feelings, and aspire to a greater command of the supernatural.

Something which has belonged to the person on whom magic is to be practised being obtained, a rag of his clothes, a nail-paring, a hair—anything so long as it is intimately connected with his personality, the magician has then that on which to work. The spittle of South Sea Island chiefs is buried in some secret place, where no sorcerer can find it, by the servants, who follow the train with spittoons; for an association, or rather sympathy of an indefinable kind, is supposed to exist between the *tubu*, as the Polynesians call it, and the person to whom it originally pertained.† The details vary in different places, but in the main the ceremony is the same everywhere. The enchanter invokes some power; it enters the *tubu*, and thence, of course, on repeated entreaty, passes naturally into the first owner of the *tubu*. When a man hears or imagines that some evil is being brought against him, it is not surprising that he should sink under his fears, or provoke the very triumph which the medicine-man has sought. Hair is nearly always required, and this illustrates and explains the nurse's dislike of bits of nails or pieces of hair not being committed to the flames at once. If a bird got any human hair, and used it for building its nest, according to a West of Scotland belief, the person whose hair had been used would become liable to headaches, and ultimately

---

* Cameron, *Across Africa*, vol i. p. 116; Oldfield, *Tr. Eth. Soc.* vol. iii. p. 246, quoted by Tylor, *Primitive Culture*, vol. i. p. 106.

† Williams, *Polynesian Researches*, vol. ii. p. 228; Lubbock, *Origin of Civilization*, p. 245; Tylor, *Early History of Mankind*, p. 129.

become bald. And why? With the light we receive from the superstitions of other nations we can look further, and see that the bold bird that used the human hair was in earlier days believed, possibly, to be an evil spirit, possibly a witch. In 1798 an image of an Indian prince was cut in wood, charmed, and buried with some of the prince's hair thrust into its side; thereupon the prince is said to have been seized by paralysis in the place in his body corresponding to the place in the image where the hair was inserted.*

When Agnes Sampson was tried she confessed that to compass the death of King James VI. of Scotland she had hung up a black toad for nine days, and collected the juice that fell from it. Had she been able to obtain a piece of linen that the king had worn she would have killed him with this venom, " causing him such extraordinarie paines as if he had beene lying upon sharpe thornes or endis of needles."†

In the island of Tauna, in the New Hebrides, Turner tells of a colony of disease-makers, who lived by collecting such rubbish as the skin of a banana which a man had eaten. The banana skin was rolled in a leaf, and slowly burned, the result being that as it burned the owner became worse and worse, and so naturally, " when a man fell sick, he knew that some sorcerer was burning his rubbish (*nahak*), and shell trumpets, which could be heard for miles were blown to signal to the sorcerers to stop and wait for the presents which would be sent next morning." ‡ The Jakun, according to the Malay, can cause sickness and death simply by beating two sticks together; it is of no consequence how far distant the house of his enemy may be, for, although the race is greatly despised, it is even more feared.

It will have been noticed that the New Hebrides sorcerers are

* Napier, *Folk-lore*, p. 114; Moor, *Hindu Pantheon*, p. 402 (note), quoted by Dalyell, *Darker Superstitions*, p. 365.
† Pitcairn, I. ii. 218; Spalding, *Elizabethan Demonology*, pp. 113, 114.
‡ Turner, *Polynesia*, pp. 18, 19, 424; Tylor, *Early History of Mankind*, p. 128.

besought to stop their incantations by blowing of trumpets, but another conception is probably involved. We can seldom be certain that the line of demarcation between cases of supernatural-origin of disease and magician-origin of disease can be pointed out, or that ravellers have grasped all the meaning of a foreign ceremony. While the discordant noise may be only a signal to the *nahak* burners to stop the burning of the banana shell, it is very possible it may have been a distinct challenge, and a recognised part of the contest between the patient and the spirit of his disease. The Stiens of Cambodia make night and day "an insupportable noise" with the view of relieving their sick from the evil influence. The Dacotas rattle gourds with beads inside and shout. The Patagonians beat drums with figures of devils painted on them at the bed of sick persons.* The following true story sent me from America by a correspondent shows the same belief in the efficacy of noise in driving away disease-demons existing among the Indians of Alaska. Captain Abram Osborne, of Edgbaston, Mass., was shipwrecked on the Alaska coast when a boy, and spent the winter among the people, who showed him and the other sailors much kindness. It happened that an old woman in the lodge where Osborne lived was suffering from a swollen face. He felt sorry for her, and made a poultice of some of the ship's bread, and with much trouble persuaded her to let him put it on. After it had been on for an hour, and no relief had been obtained, the medicine man was summoned. He came with a drum. When he beat the drum all present yelled out at the top of their voices. Louder and louder he beat, until finally he broke the drum. The patient was asked if she felt better, but as she did not a larger drum was sent for, and the beating and yelling began again. Last of all an enormous drum

---

* This beating of devils' pictures reminds us of the reasoning which induced pietists of the Middle Ages occasionally to thrash the images of those saints which had not at once answered the prayers of the faithful.

was brought with much solemnity, and more singers or criers summoned. It was in vain, for this drum was also soon broken. As the patient felt no better, a string was put about her neck, and her sufferings were ended by strangulation. It was the medical opinion of those Indians that if a disease-spirit would not be expelled by the biggest drum it could only be got rid of by destroying the body of which it had taken possession. Osborne vowed he would never again attempt the practice of medicine in a strange country. The passing bell was supposed among ourselves to drive away the evil spirits who stood waiting at the bed of the sick man for his soul. So, too, children wear bells on their clothes.*

While wizardry is sometimes hereditary, wizards, even although they escape death by the hands of their dupes, are not supposed to be always secure in their command of the supernatural. A Tauna rubbish burner sometimes discovers that an enemy is burning *his* rubbish, and blows his shells for mercy like an ordinary mortal; and of a distinguished Chinese, who, when any one in the village was ill, could point where the devils were that caused the disease and burn them out, we are told by the celestial savant, who finished his collection of stories in 1679, that before long he himself became very ill, " and his flesh turned green and purple; whereupon he said ' the devils afflict me thus because I let out their secrets. Henceforth I shall never divulge them again!' "

One of the most esteemed ways of compassing evil was to form an image of the person whose health was aimed at, and by ceremonies wreak such symbolic injury on the figure as the wizard desired in reality to fall upon the original; for, as Sir George Mackenzie puts it, " Witches do likewise torment man-

* In China children wear bells with a conciliatory purpose, because when once upon a time a rash official ordered the tabooed bell of Canton to be rung, a thousand male and female infants died within the city before the sound had died away, therefore bells are to be worn by infants that the tingle may conciliate the dreadful bell-demon.—Dennys, *Folk-lore of China*, p. 37.

kind, by making images of clay or wax, and when the witches prick or punce these images, the persons whom these images represent do find extreme torment, which doth not proceed from any influence these images have upon the body tormented, but the devil doth by natural means raise these torments in the person tormented, at the same very time that the witches do prick or punce, or hold to the fire these images of clay or wax; which manner of torment," he adds, " was lately confessed by some witches in Inverness, who likewise produced the images, and it was well known they hated the person who was tormented; and upon a confession so adminiculate, witches may very judiciously be found guilty, since *constat de corpore delicti de modo de linquendi et inimicitiis præviis.*"* Nothing is more common in the trials of the seventeenth century than such accusations against the unhappy woman who came before the court. Full details will be found in the case of Sir George Maxwell of Pollok.†

The Hindoo sorcerers attach the name of their victim to the breast of the image which is to personate him, and it is not surprising, therefore, that the Abyssinians and other peoples should conceal their baptismal name. The baptismal name is the real name, the name registered in heaven, so if the enemy who makes the image does not know this name he cannot call the image by it. If only the usual name is used, then the figure cannot properly be said to represent the original, and the danger is escaped.‡ In a Chinese tale, which tells how it was sought to discover a necromancer, the story runs that the first time the necromancer was apparently cut down, only a paper man cut through the middle was found; the second time, a clay image

* *A Treatise on Witchcraft*, 1678, § xxii.
† *Witches of Renfrewshire*, p. 43. For the conspiracy against the young laird of Fowles and the young ladie Balnagown, *see* Dalyell, p. 371.
‡ Simpson, *An Artist's Jottings in Abyssinia*, " Good Words," 1868, p. 607, " In all church services, particularly in prayers for the dead, the baptismal name must be used. How they manage to hide it I did not learn. Possibly they confide it only to the priests."

knocked to pieces; and the third time, a wooden image. The editor, in a note, says, "Taoist priests are generally credited with the power of cutting out human, animal, or other figures, of infusing vitality into them on the spot, and of employing them for purposes of good or evil."* To the employment for good, of which there are few instances, I refer elsewhere.

The most familiar way in which a personal power to cause sickness or misfortune was exercised—through what is generally known as " the evil eye "—is a subject on which so much has already been written that it is not necessary to do more here than briefly refer to it as illustrating this part of my subject. For the fact Martius vouches—" Oculis fascina induci posse, tristis experientia abunde testatur. Quamvis enim radii visini ex oculis non egrediantur, effluvia tamen emanent, quae quando livore et invidiâ malignâ redditâ per intentionem diriguntur ad certum quoddam objectum noxiam suam vim ibi exserunt."† In China, Dr. Dennys says, he has often been amused at the request not to stare at a child whose appearance had attracted him. In the early part of this century Caldcleugh speaks of a young woman being burnt, for having set evil eyes on a sick person. The Egyptian mother ascribes the sickliness of her children to the evil eye; and Arabs and Scotch Highlanders alike resort to charms against it.‡ Nor is the power efficacious against man alone; it is another instance of the belief in the close sympathy between him and nature that a Yorkshireman should be accused within this century of killing a pear tree by throwing the first glances of his evil eye in the morning upon the tree. " Look, Sir," said the informant of Mr. Carr, the compiler of *The Craven Glossary,* " at that pear-tree; it wor

* Giles, *Strange Stories from a Chinese Studio,* vol. i. pp. 49-51.
† Citing many authors.—Martius, p. 38.
‡ Dennys, *Folk-lore of China,* p. 49; Caldcleugh, *Travels* 1819-21, vol. i. p. 73; Volney, *Voyage en Syrie et en Egypte,* t. i. ch. 17, § 2, p. 223; Dalyell, *Darker Superstitions of Scotland,* p. 12. " Some persons eies are very offensive: non possum dicere quare; there is aliquid divinum in it, more than every one understands."—Aubrey, *Remains of Gentilisme* (*Folk-Lore Society's* ed.), p. 80.

some years back, Sir, a maast flourishin' tree. Ivvry mornin', as soon as he first oppans the door, *that he may not cast his e'e on onny yan passin' by*, he fixes his een o' that pear-tree, and ye plainly see how it's deed away."* The motive here was admirable. It is not long ago since an honest North Lanarkshire farmer told me of the mischief that had been caused in the dairy of a friend by a spiteful old woman. He had dismissed her son, a good-for-nothing lout, and as she, in revenge, overlooked his churn for a whole year, he was unable to get any cream. In the north of Scotland the evil eye has been said to belong to certain families, and to continue from generation to generation the inheritance which sire bequeathed to son. At the will of its possessor it was exercised not only for his private purposes of revenge but also in the service of those who paid for its exercise on their behalf against an enemy. To the present time, a correspondent writes me, the evil eye is believed in in Dorsetshire, and apart from the every day evidence afforded by newspaper cases, in which some unfortunate old woman has been maltreated, reference will often be found to some act of "overlook" which has been attributed to her. We have in the statement of the biographer of the late Vicar of Morwenstow, a proof of the hold the superstition still has in places where we should least expect to find it. Whenever Mr. Hawker came across any one with a peculiar eye-ball, sometimes bright and clear, and at other times obscured by a film, or with a double pupil ringed twice, or a larger eye to left than to right, he would adopt the ancient tactics and hold his thumb and fore and middle fingers in the peculiar position which the superstitions of Eastern Europe had taught him would ward off the evil effect of the evil eye.† Red coral was among the Romans, as among ourselves, tied round the neck of infants to protect them

---

* Carr, *Craven Glossary*, vol. i. p. 137, cited by Harland and Wilkinson, *Lancashire Folk-lore*, p. 69 (foot-note).

† Mrs. P., 30 October, 1879; Baring Gould, *Life of Rev. R. S. Hawker*, p. 152. Reference must here specially be made to the second part of Mr. Story's

from the evil eye. In Africa, Cameron found a mother who carried a baby, slung in goat-skin, on her back, wearing an apron made of innumerable thongs of hide, with a charm dangling from each, to preserve the infant from the evil eye and other forms of witchcraft. Mr. Napier, the veteran Scotch folk-lorist, says he has a vivid remembrance of having been himself considered to have got "a blink of an ill e'e" when a child. He had taken a *dwining*, which baffled the experience of his family, and to effectually remove the fascination which was working him so much ill, a neighbour "skilly" in such matters was called in. "A sixpence was borrowed from a neighbour, a good fire was kept burning in the grate, the door was locked, and I was placed upon a chair in front of the fire. The operator, an old woman, took a tablespoon and filled it with water. With the sixpence she then lifted as much salt as it could carry, and both were put into the water in the spoon. The water was then stirred with the forefinger till the salt was dissolved. Then the soles of my feet and the palms of my hands were bathed with this solution thrice, and after these bathings I was made to taste the solution three times. The operator then drew her wet forefinger across my brow, called—*scoring aboon the breath*. The remaining contents of the spoon she then cast over the fire, into the hinder part of the fire, saying, as she did so, 'Guid preserve frae a' skaith.' These were the first words permitted to be spoken during the operation. I was then put to bed, and, in attestation of the efficacy of the charm, recovered."* The scoring aboon the breath was the most common way of averting mischief. But it was more generally the

Castle of St. Angelo, which contains an exhaustive and interesting account of fascination, after which it is not necessary to go at length into the subject in these pages. *See also* Mackenzie, § xx.

* Napier, *Folk-Lore*, pp. 36, 37. Mr. Napier adds that he knows of this ceremony being performed within the last forty years, "probably in many out-lying country places it is still practised." *See* Gregor, *Folk-lore of North-East of Scotland*, p. 8.

suspected witch who was scored above the mouth, and that, unfortunately for her, with a horseshoe, till the blood came. The *Edinburgh Annual Register*, 1814, contains a notice of such a cruel act " in the upper end of Peebleshire," by a shepherd who " shrewdly suspected" that an old woman, who lived fifteen miles away, had bewitched his cows. And other instances may be found within the last fifty or sixty years.* Satan is said to have taught Jonet Irving, " if she bure ill-will to onie bodie, to look on them with *opin eyis*, and pray evil for thame in his name," " that she sould get her heartis desyre."† Martius says, surgeons do not show wounds to every man, for they have observed that by the malignant influence of some eyes healing up is of a truth hindered.‡

Foreigners, as foreigners, were naturally regarded as suspicious, and as suspicious then, allowing the simple manner of explanation which belongs to primitive peoples, likely to bring with them visible or invisible means of bringing harm on the shores on which they land. It is curious that to the present day the natives of St. Kilda should regard strangers with aversion on account of a remarkable malady, a species of influenza, locally known as " strangers' cold" (cnotan na gall), which almost invariably follows the arrival of a vessel from the outer Hebrides. The epidemic has been noticed by every writer who has visited the island, and in recent times, in 1860, when the Porcupine, commanded by Captain Otter, and having the late Duke of Athole on board, had taken its departure, in a day or two ' the trouble' made its appearance, the entire population being more or less affected by it; in 1876, when the factor's smack came, and in 1878, when the Austrian crew landed, the symptoms were as before.§ It is a curious fact, noticed by Mr. Seton, that the gradual

---

* *Edinburgh Annual Register*, 1814, chronicle portion, p. cxxxi.; Napier, *Folk-Lore*, p. 37; *Glasgow Weekly Herald*, August 5, 19, 26, 1876.
† *Trial of Jonet Irving*, 5 March, 1616; *Rec. Ork.* f. 60; Dalyell, p. 7.
‡ Martius, p. 38, quoting Joh. Agricola.
§ Seton, *St. Kilda, Past and Present*, 1878, pp. 228, 229.

extinction of certain tribes on the Amazon is said to be in great measure due to " a disease which always appears amongst them when a village is visited by people from the civilised settlements. . . . . . . The disorder has been known to break out when the visitors were entirely free from it ; the simple contact of civilised men in some mysterious way being sufficient to create it ; " and again, in the account of the cruise of H.M.S. Galatea in 1867-68, we read, " Tristan d'Acunha is a remarkably healthy island ; but it is a singular fact that any vessel touching there from St. Helena invariably brings with it a disease resembling influenza."*

(3.) That disease should be caused by the dead is not a conception which can belong to the earlier ages of culture. That death was possible was the first difficulty, and a great one, but that death could be caused by a species of warfare between the dead and the living would certainly be even as great a difficulty. To believe that the inanimate body which lay before him was not actually devoid of all the higher attributes of life would not be foreign to the reasoning of a savage, for to suppose that a single blow, a fall, or a mysterious thrust from nature, could at once and for ever cut a man off from his fellows must have been more difficult of credence ; but to fear the dying, not because they were going into an unknown country in an incomprehensible manner, but, as some peoples have said, lest a dying man who has not been parted with on friendly terms should return to wreak revenge, must be a comparatively late-born theory. It is more natural to regard the dead ancestors as beneficent minor deities than as devils,—to believe with the Tasmanians that the newly dead exercise their first spiritual powers in curing disease, and with the Malay islanders to look for prosperity and help from those who are now beyond the troubles of earth.

Not improbably the dread of the spirits of the dead in general

* Bates, *The Naturalist on the River Amazon ; Cruise of H.M.S Galatea*, cited by Mr. Seton, pp. 232, 233.

arose from dread of the spirits of the magicians in particular. Turanian tribes of North Asia, according to Castrén, fear their shamans more when they have quitted earth than when they were in the full exercise of their power on earth; the Patagonians have no doubt of the evil demons who afflict their lives being the spirits of dead wizards.* But this fear of particular spirits soon developed. The Chinese have a general dislike of spirits of lepers, beggars, and other outcasts. " Selon les Tchérémisses," Hexthausen (quoted by Lenormant) says, "les âmes des morts viennent inquiéter les vivants, et, pour les en empêcher, ils percent la plante des pieds et le cœur des morts, convaincus que, cloués ainsi dans leur tombe, ils n'en pourront sortir." †

In Madagascar, among the Sàkàlava, when a death occurs in one of their villages, the settlement is broken up, and the tribe remove their homes some distance from their former abode, believing that the spirits of the dead will haunt the spot, and do harm to those who remain in the place where it had dwelt.‡ Mr. Conway says that in 1875 he was told by an eminent physician of Chicago, whose name he gives, of a case which, within his personal knowledge, had occurred in that city, in which the body of a woman, who had died of consumption, was taken out of the grave and the lungs burned, under the belief that she was drawing after her into the grave some of her surviving relatives; and he also quotes an account of a Mr. Rose, of Peacedale, Rhode Island, who in the previous year dug up the body of his own daughter, and burned her heart, because, it was believed, she was wasting away the lives of other members of his family. The people of Morzine, in Savoy, in 1857,

---

* Castrén, *Finn Myth.*, p. 122; Falkner, *Patagonia*, p. 116; Tylor, *Primitive Culture*, vol. ii. p. 102 (see also vol. ii. p. 175).

† Doolittle, *Chinese*, vol. i. p. 206; Hexthausen, *Études sur la situation intérieure de la Russie*, t. i. p. 419; Lenormant, *La Magie chez les Chaldéens*, pp. 187, 188; *Folk-Lore Record*, vol. ii. p. 41. Vampire stories are also illustrative of this superstition.

believed themselves to be actually possessed by the spirits of dead persons whilst they suffered the epidemic called hysterodemonapathy.* The natives of the Transvaal, after mutilating, roasting, and partially eating the body of an enemy, mix blood and clay and smear their faces with the mixture in order to protect them from the revenge of the spirit of the man who has been killed. Their regard for the influence of the dead is manifested in many ways. Medicine poured into the wounds of the dead son of a chief would, it was believed, cause the death of those who had killed him, and this seems to be a general practice. The Polynesians speak of departed souls devouring the hearts and entrails of sleepers.†

Among ourselves, it is a Devonshire belief that you can give a neighbour ague by burying a dead man's hair under his threshold. Passing over a hidden grave was said, in Aberdeenshire, to produce a rash. In New Jersey, it is said to cause incurable cramps in the foot. If any article from one's person, such as a pin, be buried with a corpse, the man or woman to whom it belonged will also be with the dead before the year is out. Ulster men also speak of *dead men's pinches*, small discoloured marks on the skin, resembling pinches or bruises, which come in the night in some mysterious way.‡

In olden England such proceedings mentioned above as having taken place in America would not have been permitted, for it was believed that to exhume any body would be an act followed by death and calamity in the deceased's family, as the following illustrates :—

* Conway, *Demonology and Devil-Lore*, vol. i. p. 52 ; *Cornhill Magazine*, April 1865, " The Devils of Morzine."

† *Christian Express* (South Africa), January, 1879, " Transvaalia," by Rev. A. Kropf, p. 8 ; Tylor, *Primitive Culture*, vol. ii. p. 175.

‡ Gregor, *Folk-lore of North-East of Scotland*, p. 35 ; Miss G. (Rochester, U.S.A.), 28 November, 1879 ; W. H. P. (Belfast), 26 October, 1878. Among the charms found by Mr. Ellis in the basket laid at his door and designed to bring evil were " hedgehog's bristles, parts of scorpions or centipedes, hair, earth said to be from a grave," &c. *Madagascar Revisited*, p. 271; *Folk-Lore Record*, vol. ii. p. 43.

"Thomas Fludd, of Kent, Esq., told me that it is an old observation which was pressed earnestly to King James I. that he should not remove the Queen of Scots' body from Northamptonshire, where she was beheaded and interred. For that it always bodes ill to the family when bodies are removed from their graves, for some of the family will die shortly after, as did Prince Henry, and I think Queen Anne."*

The belief that the dead cause the diseases of the living is strikingly shown in the inhuman dislike manifested alike in China and Scotland to save a drowning man. The government of Hong-Kong has found it necessary to insert a clause in the junk clearances, binding the junkmen to assist to the utmost in saving life. The theory of the Chinese is that the spirits of persons who have died a violent death, may return to earth if they can find a substitute. Thus, if A has just lost his son B, and is mourning his loss, should he see C struggling in the water he naturally will not help him,—he would rather see him quickly drowned, for so will B return to life all the sooner. As for C, it is his fate, and he has only to wait until another person— D, E, or F—comes to the same end. The last man dead is supposed to keep watch and ward over the land of the dead; to save a drowning man would be to defraud him of his substitute, and to incur the serious displeasure of a mysterious enemy.†

Mr. Tylor regards the dislike manifested by the Hindoo, who will not save a man from drowning in the sacred Ganges, the Malay, the Kamchadal, the Bohemian, and other peoples, as indicating a universal belief that to snatch a victim from the very clutches of the water-spirit is a rash defiance of deity which would hardly pass unavenged.‡ He regards the drowning man as an offering to the spirit of the sea, or river, or lake; a spirit

* Turner, *History of the Most Remarkable Providences*, Lond. 1677, p. 77, cited in *Notes and Queries*, 1st S. vol. ii. p. 4.
† Dennys, *Folk-Lore of China*, p. 22; see also Giles, *Strange Stories from a Chinese Studio*, vol. ii. p. 200.
‡ Tylor, *Primitive Culture*, vol. i. pp. 97-99.

which, if not propitiated in some such manner, will necessarily take revenge in some more terrible way. But although this explanation may be regarded as sufficient in some cases, I cannot regard it as applicable to all these illustrations of the prejudice. On the contrary, the remarkable similarity between the Chinese and the Celtic theories lead me to believe that the conception of a water-deity, who must be duly regaled with sacrifice, is generally subordinate to the belief that the soul of the last dead man is insulted, or done injustice to, by preventing another from taking his place.

The Scotch did not regard the last death of so much consequence as the last burial. "The spirit of the last person buried watches round the churchyard till another is buried, to whom he delivers his charges."* "It was the duty of the last person interred to stand sentry at the graveyard gate from sunset until the crowing of the cock every night until regularly relieved. This sometimes, in thinly-inhabited parts of the country, happening to be a tedious and severe duty, and the duration of the *faire claidth* gave the deceased's surviving friends much uneasiness." The idea that the spirit had to watch the graveyard is a distinctly lower conception than that of the Chinese, who regard him as sentry in the unseen world, and is probably of late and explanatory introduction. Still, we can see clearly why Bryce, the pedlar in Sir Walter Scott's *Pirate*, refused to aid Mordaunt in saving the sailor from drowning, "Are you mad," he said, "you that have lived sae lang in Zetland, to risk the saving of a drowning man." It is true, he adds, "Wat ye not, if you bring him to life again, he will be sure to do you some capital injury?" But it should be remembered that the Celts were not strangers to a doctrine of possession, and it is easy to imagine that the defrauded spirit on guard, when he at last procured his release, should take the first oppor-

* *New Statistical Account of Scotland*, vol. xiv. p. 210.

tunity of inflicting injury on him who had prevented the shortening of his term, and that most readily through the very man who should have been the substitute.

So terrible was the question, that we hear in Scotland, in the last century, of quarrels as to who should be first buried in the churchyard. In one case, when two burials were appointed for one day, "both parties staggered forward as fast as possible to consign their respective friend in the first place in the dust." If they met at the gate, the dead were thrown aside until the living decided by blows whose ghost should be condemned to porter it.* In October, 1876, two men, residing outside of Nenagh, Tipperary, were accidentally drowned together through the upsetting of a cart, in which they were crossing a small river. At the funeral a free fight took place between the two parties of friends, each desiring that its corpse should be the first to enter the graveyard, since it was believed that the last buried would have to act as servitor to the other (*i.e.* the *faire claidth* of the Scotch). Mr. Napier's suggestion, that the spirit watched "lest any suicide or unbaptised child should be buried in consecrated ground,"† is a modern engraftment, an attempt to explain a tradition of great antiquity in accordance with more modern teachings.

Among miscellaneous theories to account for diseases or illnesses we note that in Ulster the brown foam from the seashore is said to cause warts to grow ; and as warts are said in Ulster always to come in pairs, a wart on the thumb of the right hand being balanced by a wart on the thumb of the left hand, care should evidently be taken. So, too, if one treads on hungry grass—which is said to grow up where persons dining in a field have not thrown some of the fragments to the fairies— he will be seized with what the Irish call *feargartha* or *fairgurtha*, hungry disease, an intolerable hunger and weakness.‡

* *New Statistical Account of Scotland*, vol. xxi. p. 114.
† *Folk-lore of the West of Scotland*, p. 63.
‡ W. H. P. (Belfast), 26 October, 1878 ; *Folk-Lore Record*, vol. iv. p. 109.

Harelip, in the north-east of Scotland, is said to be produced by a woman *enceinte* putting her foot into a hare's lair. If a woman discovers she has done this she should put two stones in the lair. Cancer was supposed to be produced by the bite of a pig, but soup made of fresh pork, as "pork bree," was looked upon as efficacious in the highest degree in cases of consumption or dyspepsia.* Killing a toad is said in New England to have the undesirable result of ensuring its slaughterer as many warts as it had spots. Vermont people add that such an act dries up the cows.†

The Chinese sometimes attribute disease to the absence of the spirit, and in the case of a little child lying dangerously ill, Mr. Giles says its mother will go outside into the garden and call its name several times in the hope of bringing back the wandering spirit.‡

Disease is brought upon men at St. Elian's Well, parish of Llanelian, Denbighshire, by casting a pin along with a pebble marked with the victim's initials into the well. The person cursed soon hears of the cruel charm, and it is not surprising that, ruminating upon all the forms of disease to which it may be possible that he will be doomed, should readily induce, if not an actual sickness in a healthy man, at least a craving for the removal of the impending curse. It is easily removed; the pebble is taken out, the name is removed from the magician's book, and, once more free from the fear of the powers of this unholy well, the thankful spared can go about his work with lightened heart.§

A mysterious sympathy is sometimes supposed to exist between men and natural objects. Thus, when children have been passed through cleft trees (a ceremonial to which more detailed

* Gregor, *Folk-lore of North-East of Scotland*, p. 129, but compare Nork, *Mythologie der Volkssagen, &c.*, p. 322.
† Miss C. G. (Rochester, N.Y.), 28 November, 1879.
‡ Giles, *Strange Stories*, vol. i. p. 189.
§ Wirt Sykes, *British Goblins*, pp. 355-6.

reference will be found later on), the child's life is supposed in a manner to be bound up with that of the particular tree through which he has been transmitted, and, should an attempt be unadvisedly made to cut the tree, no efforts will be spared by the man to secure the continued existence of his foster-brother. In the reign of Romanus Lacapenus it was desirable that Simeon, Prince of Bulgaria, should die. Now, on the arch Xerolophi, in Constantinople, there stood a column, and an astronomer assured Romanus that if the head of this column were struck off, Simeon, whose fate was bound up with it, would perish. The head was accordingly struck from the pillar, and at the same hour on the same day the prince died in Bulgaria of a disease of the heart.*

The wide-spread belief that toothache is caused by a worm in the offending tooth is not a little curious. In 1607 an English version of the *Regimen Sanitatis Salernitanum* of the eleventh century says:—

> "If in your teeth you hap to be tormented
>   By meane some little wormes therein do breed,
> Which pain (if need be tane) may be prevented,
>   Be keeping cleane your teeth, when as you feede;
> Burne Francomsence (a gum not evil sented),
>   Put Henbane unto this, and Onyon seed,
> And with a tunnel to the tooth that's hollow,
> Convey the smoke thereof, and ease shall follow." †

Only four years ago a person of considerable education told me how the worm had been removed from his tooth nine years previously by a Greenock working-man. The method was exactly the same, but it is scarcely necessary to say frankincense

---

* Cedrenus, *Compendium Historiarum*, t. ii. p. 625, cited in Dalyell's *Darker Superstitions of Scotland*, pp. 365, 366.

† "The Englishman's Doctor; or, the School of Salerne," *Notes and Queries*, 5th S. vol. vi. p. 97. The Latin runs,

> "Sic dentes serva, porrorum collige grana,
> Ne careas jure (thure?) cum hyoscyamo ure,
> Sicque per embotum fumum cape dente remotum."
> Vv. 240-2.

was not used. My impression is that tobacco was resorted to instead. Shakspeare, in *Much Ado About Nothing*, mentions the belief: "What!" says Don Pedro, "sign for the toothache?" "Where is," says Leonato, "but a humour or a worm." In Aberdeenshire, in China, in Orkney, in New Zealand, in Derbyshire, in North Germany, everywhere one might almost say, this belief is found. In Madagascar the sufferer from toothache is described as being *maràry olitra* (poorly through the worm). In Manx the plural form of *Beisht* (a beast), *Beishtyn*, is used for the toothache, "from the opinion that the pain arose from an animal in the tooth," and in Gaelic *cnuimh*, a worm, gives half the name of toothache, which is *cnuimh fhiacall.** The remedies for "toothworms" given in the first Leech Book are quaint:—

"For toothwark, if a worm eat the tooth, take an old holly leaf or one of the lower umbels of hart wort, and the upward part of sage, boil two doles (*i.e.* two of worts to one of water) in water, pour into a bowl and yawn over it, then the worms shall fall into the bowl.

"If a worm eat the teeth, take holly rind over a year old and root of carline thistle, boil in hot water, hold in the mouth as hot as thou hottest may.

"For tooth worms, take acorn meal and henbane seed and wax, of all equally much, mingle these together, work into a wax candle and burn it, let it reek into the mouth, put a black cloth under, then will the worms fall on it."† In Norfolk one would think such ceremonies must be unknown if, as some say, toothache is called the love pain there, and sufferers consequently receive little sympathy.

* *Choice Notes* (*Folk-Lore*), p. 62 ; *Notes and Queries*, 5th S. vol. v. pp. 24, 155, 476; vol. vi. p. 97 ; *Folk-Lore Record*, vol. ii. p. 36 ; Kelly, *Manx Dictionary*; McLeod and Dewar, *Gaelic Dictionary*; Shortland, *Traditions and Superstitions of the New Zealanders*, pp. 108-110.

† Cockayne, *Saxon Leechdoms*, vol. ii. p. 51. For instances of this superstition, see also *Derbyshire Gatherer*, p. 204.

CHAPTER II.

TRANSFERENCE OF DISEASE.

WHEN disease was recognised, though tardily, to have positive existence, and the fact realised that, despite prayers and offerings, it might mysteriously be communicated by the sick man to another person who suffered in much the same way, complaining of similar pains and exhibiting the same general symptoms, a step had been taken in folk-medicine. If a man could without conscious act on his part infect his neighbours, why might he not *of purpose* transfer his complaint to something of a lower order, which should suffer the disease in his place?* This is a specious reasoning, and may not unreasonably be supposed to have found early acceptance. Since powers beyond the reach of man were able to give a particular disease to every sufferer; since those powers settled in the person of a witch or a medicine man enabled them to transfer one creature's distemper to another; was it not possible that an ordinary human being should be able at least to transfer disease to a slave, a dog, or a horse? Pliny speaks of pains in the stomach being cured by transferring the ailment into a puppy or a duck.† To inhale the cold breath of a duck

---

* " Per quam Naturæ peritus morbum mediis licitis ex homine aliorsum transfert, ut sanitas exinde sequatur."—Martius, p. 27.

† " Sunt occulti interaneorum morbi, de quibus mirum proditur. Si catuli, priusquam videant, applicentur triduo stomacho maxime ac pectori et ex ore aegri suctum lactis accipiant, transire vim morbi, postremo exanimari dissectisque palam fieri aegri causas." " Quod praeterea traditur in torminibus mirum est, anate apposita ventri transire morbum anatemque emori."—Pliny, 30, 7. " So hat man noch bis in den letzten jahrhunderten junge welfe angelegt und saugen lassen."—Grimm, *Deutsche Mythologie*, vol. ii. p. 980. See also vol. iii. p. 343.

is still recommended in England. In Devonshire and in Scotland alike when a child has whooping-cough a hair is taken from its head, put between slices of bread and butter, and given to a dog, and if in eating it the dog cough—as naturally he will—the whooping-cough will be transferred to the animal, and the child will go free. Indeed this remedy is practised with local variation all over the country. In some parts of Ireland when one has been attacked with scarlet fever some of the sick man's hair is cut off, and passed down the throat of an ass, which is supposed then and there to receive the illness. Ague in a boy is cured by a cake made of barley-meal and his urine and given to a dog to eat; the dog in a case cited had a shaking fit, and the boy was cured!*

Possibly the simplest mode of transference is given by Pierius; the patient is to sit on an ass, with his face to the tail, and thus the pain will be transmitted to the ass.†

Marcellus, of old, to cure toothache recommended the patient to spit in a frog's mouth, and request him to make off with the toothache, and in Cheshire it is still by no means uncommon for a young frog to be held for a few moments with its head inside the mouth of a sufferer from aptha or thrush. The frog is supposed to become the recipient of the ailment, which has, indeed, in some districts received the folk-name of " the frog " from the association. " I assure you," said an old Shropshire woman as she finished her account of the cure which she had often superintended, " we used to hear the poor frog whooping and coughing, mortal bad, for days after; it would have made your heart

---

* Pettigrew, *Superstitions connected with the Practice of Medicine and Surgery*, p. 77. Madame de Scudery mentions a similar cure for fever in a letter of date 20 October, 1677, to the Comte de Bussy. Speaking of an abbé of fame, " On dit qu'il ne fait que prendre pour toutes fièvres de l'urine des malades dans laquelle il fait durcir un œuf hors de sa coque, apres quoi il le donne à manger à un chien qui prend en même tems la fièvre du malade, qui par ce moien en guerit. C'est un question de fait que je n'ay pas éprouvé."—*Notes and Queries*, 5th S. vol. viii. p. 126.

† Pettigrew, p. 78.

ache to hear the poor creature coughing as it did about the garden." *

Toads are also used in cases of whooping-cough, but fish are occasionally substituted, as the following shows:—" An old fisherman, formerly well-known at the Forge, Keswick, once caught a fish, which he put into the mouth of a child suffering from whooping-cough. He then replaced the fish in the Grata. He affirmed that the fish, after being placed in the mouth of the child and returned to the river, gave the complaint to the rest of its kind, as was evident from the fact that they came to the top to cough." Apart from old Edmundson's fable, it is clear that the superstition did exist in Cumberland. Mr. Henderson also refers to it, and to a correspondent of *Notes and Queries* we are indebted for an account of the practice in America : " One morning, during the early fall of the present year (1875)," he says, " I was wandering along the banks of the Schuylkill river, in the neighbourhood of Philadelphia. The day being sultry, I sat down on a projecting rock to enjoy the cool breeze from the water. Near by stood two men fishing with rod and line. Presently a young woman, carrying a child some two years old, made her appearance, and, approaching one of the anglers, asked him for a fish he had just caught. Americans, as a rule, are extremely courteous to the gentler sex, so, taking it from the hook, he politely handed it to her, when, seating herself on the bank, she deliberately opened the child's mouth, and, thrusting in the head of the fish, held it there, despite the child's struggles, for the space of a minute or two, then, withdrawing it she consigned the still living animal to its native element. My curiosity being aroused by this rather novel proceeding, I requested an explanation, when she informed me that the child was afflicted with the whooping-cough, and that the head of a living fish held

* Cockayne, *Leechdoms*, vol. i. p. xxx.; *Jour. Brit. Arch. Assoc.* vol. xxxiv. p. 328; W. H. 7 September, 1880; Rev. G. S. S. 24 November, 1878.

for a moment in the sufferer's mouth was 'a sure and certain' cure for that complaint." The writer was unable to tell from what nation this custom had been derived as the population was of very mixed descent.*

Marcellus distinguished between six kinds of transference or transplantation: (a) inseminatione; (b) implantatione; (c) impositione; (d) irritatione; (e) inescatione; (f) adproximatione; but in practical folk-medicine the method followed is always the same. The creature to be infected is brought into immediate contact with the suffering person, and, after time allowed for ordinary infection, is set free.

Sometimes, however, the disease is only intended to be a temporary burden. Thus Steinhauser, speaking of the custom, in West Africa, of transferring a sick man's ailment to a live fowl, says if any one catches the fowl when set free the disease goes to him, and incidental illustrations of this case will be found in many cases of transference.

Transference to inanimate objects is not uncommon. In development of the original theory Salmuth relates a case of cure by transplantation. The patient had a most violent pain of the arm, and "they beat up red coral with oaken leaves, and, having kept them on the part affected till suppuration, they did in the morning put this mixture into an hole bored with an augur in the root of an oak, respecting the east, and stopt up this hole with a peg, made of the same tree; from thenceforth the pain did altogether cease, and when they took out the amulet, immediately the torments returned sharper than before." Grimm has several notes on this subject. "Beachtenswerth," he says, "ist dies übertragen der krankheit auf bäume, d.h. auf den geist, der in ihnen wohnt. Unten den beschwörungsformeln beginnt xxvi. mit den worten: 'zweig ich biege dich, fieber nun lass mich!'

---

* *Notes and Queries,* 5th S. vol. ix. p. 64; vol. iii. p. 345; see also Henderson's *Folk-Lore of the Northern Counties,* p. 141.

'Hollerast hebe dich auf, rothlauf setze dich drauf, ich hab dich einen tag, habe dus jahr und tag.'" He who has gout goes on three successive Fridays after sunset to a fir tree, and says, "Tannenbaum, ich klage dir, die gicht plagt mich schier," and so on,—the fir will wither, and the gout disappear. "Deus vos salvet sambuce, panem et sal ego vobis adduca, febrem tertianam et quotidianam accipiatis vos, qui nolo eam."* Westendorp, quoted by Grimm, gives the following Dutch charm for a fever: The patient must go at the break of day to an old willow, tie three notes on a branch of it, and say, "Goe morgen, olde, ik geef oe de kolde, goe morgen olde." Then he turns and runs without looking back.† A similar New England charm for an obstinate ague has been sent to me by an American correspondent. The patient in this case is to take a string made of woollen yarn, of three colours, and to go by himself to an apple tree; there he is to tie his left hand loosely with the right to the tree by the tricoloured string, then to slip his hand out of the knot, and run into the house without looking behind him.‡ In Cheshire the absolute transference of warts is worth noting. Steal a piece of bacon and rub the warts with it, then cut a slit in the bark of an ash tree, and slip in the bacon under a piece of the bark. Speedily the warts will disappear from the hand, but will make their appearance on the bark of the tree as rough excrescences, and the success of this remedy has been vouched for.§

Martius speaks of piercing the gums in case of toothache, "dum sanguinem fundant," with a piece of bark, then returning the bark, covered as it will be with blood, to the tree, and covering it carefully with mud. "Et corticem reductum luto

* Boyle, *Usefulness of Experimental Philosophy*, pp. 226, 227; Pettigrew, p. 77; Grimm, *Deutsche Mythologie*, vol. ii. p. 979.

† A common prohibition, see *Herbarium Apuleii;* Cockayne, *Leechdoms*, vol. i. p. 99.

‡ Miss C. F. G. (Rochester, U.S A.), 28 November, 1879.

§ *Science Gossip*, 1865, p. 85; *Folk-Lore Record*, vol. i. p. 158.

bene muni." This, he avows, is useful in cases of habitual or constantly recurring toothache.* Sir Kenelm Digby for toothache directs the gum to be cut with an iron nail till it bleed, and then the nail with blood upon it is to be driven into a wooden beam up to the head. When this is done, you never shall have toothache again all your days. Within the last forty years there was a charmer in Riccarton, near Kilmarnock, who cured toothache after this fashion, but more simply. He did not put his patients to further pain by scarifying the gum with the nail; he only drove a nail into the beam which supported the roof of his house. In course of time it became studded with nails, from the fact that possibly the beams first so employed were of oak; some say that to drive a nail into an oak tree is sufficient to cure toothache.

Certain oak trees at Berkhampstead, in Hertfordshire, were long famous for the cure of ague. The transference was simple but painful. A lock of hair was pegged into an oak, and then by a sudden wrench transferred from the head of the patient to the tree.

Mr. Tylor, on the authority of Mr. Spottiswoode, says:—" In Thuringia it is considered that a string of rowan berries, a rag, or any small article touched by a sick person, and then hung on a bush beside some forest path, imparts the malady to any person who may touch this article in passing, and frees the sick man from the disease. This gives great probability to Captain Burton's suggestion that the rags, locks of hair, and what not hung on trees near sacred places by the superstitious, from Mexico to India, and Ethiopia to Ireland, are deposited there as actual receptacles for transference of disease."† An Irish instance immediately suggests itself. At the holy well, Tubber Quan, near Carrick-on-Suir, the faithful were (and for all we

---

* Martius, *De Magia*, p. 32; Cf. Daniel Beceri, *Microcosm. Med.* lib. i. c. 14, pp. 75, *et seq.*

† Tylor, *Primitive Culture*, vol. ii. p. 187.

know are) wont to resort on the three last Sundays in June to pray to St. Quan and St. Brogaum, who, if cures are to be vouchsafed, appear in the holy well in the shape of two wondrously fair trout. After the pilgrims have gone through some trying penances, they cut locks of their hair, and tie them on the branches of a certain tree (round which they have three times gone on their bare knees) as specifics, so the account runs, against headaches. "The tree is a great object of veneration, and presents a curious spectacle, being covered all over with human hair." The Dayacks, with a feeling akin, hang rags on the trees at crossways. In Malabar, the practice reminds us of the trees at Berkhampstead, but in this case the patient is securely tied to the tree, and flogged before his hair is fastened in. This has been cited as an instance "that hair may be a substitute for its owner," but I think it may also be looked upon as belonging to transference. Morier* presents us with an essential modification of the theory. In Persia, according to his account, the patient has only to deposit a rag on certain bushes, and from the same spot to take another, which has been left there from the same motives by a previous visitor and sufferer. This is a further development of the theory, but not one, apparently, which took such firm hold of the European mind. The Persian custom, considered by itself, would probably suggest that the rags and other things were offerings to tree-spirits, and this is a conception which should be kept in view. The Persian theory may be that by offering the rag, or other article, the patient is cured, without involving evil consequences to the next person who touches it. The fact of offering may presume purification, and the next pilgrim takes with him a sanctified charm. Captain Burton speaks of articles into which spirits had been drawn being driven into or hung to a devil's tree, and this "has the effect of laying the disease spirit." A subtler reasoning, but of the

* *Journey to Persia*, p. 230.

same nature, may perhaps serve to elucidate the custom mentioned by Morier.

In Scotland, John Dougall was libelled on November 12, 1695, for having, among other things, prescribed as a cure for convulsions parings from the sick man's nails, and hair from his eyebrows, and the crown of his head "bound up in a clout, with a halfpenny," which should be laid down in a certain place, and that whoever found would take the disease, and the diseased be set free.* In Germany, an offensive form of transference also exists, for a plaster from a sore, if left at a crossway, is believed to transfer the disease to a passer-by. In Ireland, a correspondent informs me, if a charm or a curse is left on a gate or stile, the first healthy person who passes through will have the patient's sickness transferred to him.† Here there is no mention made of either the charm being in contact with the patient, and thus acquiring the disease, or of the newly-infected having even touched the dangerous paper. It is enough that the charm has a potency of its own, great enough to render the gate or passage to which it is attached, and which is between it and the passer-by, an actual source of disease.

The most common mode of transference in this country requires a short notice. Lancashire wise men tell us—" for warts rub them with a cinder, and this tied up in paper, and dropped where four roads meet (*i.e.* where the roads cross), will transfer the warts to whoever opens the parcel." Another mode of transferring warts is to touch each wart with a pebble, and place the pebbles in a bag, which should be lost on the way to church; whoever finds the bag gets the warts. Hunt says that a Cornish lady told him that when a child, out of curiosity, and in ignorance, she once took up such a bag, and examined its contents, the lamentable consequence being that in a short time she had as many warts as there were stones in the bag. A Scottish

* Vide *Witches of Renfrewshire*, p. xxiii.
† W. H. P. (Belfast), 6 November, 1878.

version bids the sufferer wrap up in a parcel as many grains of barley as there are warts, and lay the parcel on the public road. Whoever finds and opens it receives the warts. A still simpler plan is to go to a point where four roads meet, lift a stone, rub the warts with the dust from below the stone, repeating the words—

"A'm ane, the wart's twa,
The first ane it comes by
Tacks the warts awa'."

The warts will soon vanish.* In Shetland a person affected with ringworm takes on three successive mornings ashes between the forefinger and thumb, before taking food, and, while holding them to the part affected, says—

"Ringworm, ringworm red!
Never mayst thou spread or speed
But aye grow less and less
And die away among the ase (*ashes*).†

There seems here no intention of transferring the ringworm to any other person, but simply that the ashes may in some way receive and dispose of the disease, as in South Lincolnshire, when warts have been rubbed nine times with an apple cut into nine pieces, the sections are reunited, are not left abroad for the unwary, but buried where no human foot treads.‡

Boys in some parts of the United States revert to the unfortunate toad for the cure of their warts, rubbing them against one of those unfortunate creatures impaled on a sharp stick.§

A curious mode of getting clear of disease is by forcing it in some manner upon the dead. A charm for boils consists in poulticing the boil for three days and nights, and then placing the poultices, and their cloths, in the coffin of a dead man.‖ So, too,

* Harland and Wilkinson, *Lancashire Folk-Lore*, p. 157; Hunt, *Romances and Drolls*, second series, p. 211; Gregor, *Folk-Lore of North-East of Scotland*, p. 48.
† *Choice Notes* (*Folk-Lore*), p. 38.
‡ But this possibly from a sympathetic feeling, that as the apple decays the warts will go.
§ Wirt Sikes, *British Goblins*, p. 352.
‖ Dyer, *English Folk-Lore*, p. 171.

in the case of rheumatism in Donegal. I cannot do better than quote the picturesque account of the scene given by a recent writer. " At a wake in Fannet, a wild region on the Donegal coast, a man bent almost double, and tottering slowly, supported by his stick, entered the house, and sat down by the fire. He was a neighbour of the bereaved family, so that the people smoking round the hearth in the ' wake-house ' were not surprised to see him join them. It was the day of the funeral; the coffin had arrived, and the dead man was about to be laid within it, and carried to his long rest. But before they raised him from the bed, the cripple man crept over, and taking the hand of the corpse, applied it to his arm, to his shoulder, and to his leg, saying, ' Tak' my pains wi' you, Thady, in the name of God!' The neighbours and family stepped back, whispering, ' Poor Donald! poor crayther, he's sore afflicted wi' the pains, why shouldn't he try the cure?' Again, when the coffin was being lifted over the threshold, Donald called after it, ' Tak' my pains wi' you, Thady, in the name of God?' ' Was the cure successful?' we asked our informant. 'Ay, Donald threw away the stick, an' walked as weel's I do; but sure, miss dear, it was a harsh unfeeling thing to do. I'd sooner ha' suffered the pains.' Donald, who tried the cure, and Kitty, who told us of it, are Roman Catholics, and their idea probably was that the pains of rheumatism would be an imperceptible addition to those of Purgatory."* Whether the fair folklorist is right in her final surmise or not there can be little doubt of the approval with which such conveyance to the dead has been received. In Kent, if a man wets his forefinger with saliva, and rubs the wart he wishes to get rid of three times in the same direction as a passing funeral, saying each time (without any of the ceremony above observed) " My wart goes with you," a cure will soon follow.† In Donegal, the words are preceded by throwing a stone after the corpse in the

* " Fairy Superstitions in Donegal," *Univ. Mag.* Aug. 1879, pp. 214, 215.
† Dyer, *English Folk-Lore*, p. 167.

name of the Father, the Son, and the Holy Ghost.* There, too, only the corpse of a person who has no near relative or "sib" is to be so treated. The custom of burying pins which have touched warts in a newly-made grave seems to belong to this belief. They are generally placed in a bottle; the remedy is considered infallible.†

But the transference of disease was not always a simple voluntary act on the part of the patient; on the contrary, in Scotland it became a work which demanded the energies of the best reputed witches. Thus Agnes Sampson, who was tried for witchcraft in 1590, had been called in to cure Robert Kerr of a disease "laid on him be ane Westland warloc quhen he was at Dumfries, quhilk seiknes sche tuck vpone hirself, and keipit the samen with grit greiving and torment quhill the morne," when she naturally tried to transfer it by some clothes to a cat or a dog, and "thair wes ane grit dyn hard in the haus." By some mistake, however, the disease was transferred to Alexander Douglas, of Dalkeith, who pined away and died thereof, while Robert Kerr "was maid haill."‡

When Margaret Hutchinson was charged with transferring a disease from a woman to a cat, it was urged in her defence that the argument was not relevant because Sir George Mackensie notes, it was said, (1), una saga non potest esse ligans et solvens in eodem morbo (the same witch cannot both cause and cure a disease); (2), that in such transactions as these, the devil never used to interpose his skill, except where he was a gainer; and therefore, though he would transfer a disease from a brute to a rational creature, yet he would never transfer a disease from a rational creature to a beast, but these defences were repelled, since, as the devil could make sick and make whole, it followed that he could also transfer disease as he pleased.

* *Border Mag.* August, 1863, "Wart and Wen Cures," and *Folk-Lore Record*, vol. i. p. 223. See also *Choice Notes (Folk-Lore)*, p. 251; Aubrey, p. 118.
† Hunt, *Romances and Drolls*, second series, p. 210.
‡ Dalyell, *Darker Superstitions of Scotland*, pp. 104, 105.

Katherine Grieve cured Elspeth Tailyeour of a deadly disease by transferring it to a calf, which immediately died. So too another woman, also in the seventeenth century, was cured by the transference of her disease to a cow, which "ran woid and deit"; and other instances of alleged transference to a mare, to a lamb, to a cat, to a dog, may be found in the witch prosecutions of the time.

One instance given by Dalyell, although he does not seem to regard it as belonging to transference, is too remarkable not to be quoted: " The accusation of Marioun Ritchart, ' Ye cam to Stronsay, and asking almes of Andro Coupar, skipper of ane bark;' he said, ' Away witch, carling; devil ane farthing ye will fall ! ' quhairvpoun ye went away verie offendit, and incontinentlie, he going to sea, the bark being vnder saill, he rane wode, and wald have luppen (leapt) ourboord; and his sone seeing him, gat him in armes, and held him; quhairvpon the seiknes immediatelie left him, and his sone ran wode; and Thomas Paiterson seeing him tak his madness, *and the father to turn weill*, ane dog being in the bark, took the dog, and bladdit [struck] him vpon the tua schoulderis, and thairefter flang the said dogg in the sea, quhairby these in the bark were saiffed.' " Nothing could be clearer than this. The madness of the father at once communicated itself to the son, and the son's madness in turn was communicated by the careful Thomas Paiterson to the dog. The dog's death at once removed danger of any new infection. It does not seem to have been a case of pure oblation, and, even if this were Paiterson's idea, at least the sudden infection of the son is worthy of note in anything which deals with the transference of disease ; besides, the Shetland records inform us that transference could be effected simply by wishes, and grasping the hand of the intended sufferer.

The Hottentots in Kat River settlement, on the Eastern frontier of Cape Colony, according to a correspondent of *Notes and Queries*, in order to cure the bite of a snake, pluck a few feathers from the breast of a fowl, and make a small incision in the skin, to which the wound is applied; after some time the process is repeated, the fowl in the meantime gradually dying as the poison extracted from the wound operates on it. A somewhat similar mode of cure is practised in Devonshire,* but here civilisation has so far advanced claims to humanity that the chicken is killed, and the wound is then only thrust into its stomach, there to remain until the bird becomes cold. " If the flesh of the bird, when cold, assumes a dark colour it is believed that the cure is effected, and that the virus has been extracted from the sufferer; if, however, the flesh retains its natural colour, then the poison has been absorbed into the system of the bitten person."

Transference in Wales is a very serious ceremony, as the following account of the various observances which an epileptic patient has to go through at St. Tegla's Well, halfway between Wrexham and Ruthin, shows. The patient repairs to the well after sunset, and washes himself in it; then, having made an offering by throwing into the water fourpence, he walks round it three times, and thrice recites the Lord's Prayer. If the patient is a man, a cock is carried in a basket first round the well, then round the church, and if a woman, a hen is substituted. The paternoster is again repeated, and the patient then enters the church, creeps under the altar and remains there until break of day, with the Bible for pillow. In the morning another offering, this time of sixpence, is made, and the cock or hen left in the church. Should the bird die, it is supposed that the disease has been transferred to it, and the man or woman consequently cured.† In 1855 the parish clerk of Llandegla, says Mr. Sikes, said that an old man of his acquaintance remembered quite well seeing the birds staggering about from the effects of the fits which had been transferred to them.‡

* Dyer, *English Folk-Lore*, p. 137.
† *Arch. Camb.* first series, vol. i. p. 184, quoted in *British Goblins*, p. 329.
‡ Wirt Sikes, *British Goblins*, p. 350.

Animal diseases were likewise transferred; and of this practice we have, as might be expected, more instances in the last two or three hundred years than of transference of men's diseases. The animal who had died of plague, or some other serious disorder, was carried at night to a neighbouring proprietor's land and buried—sometimes in a wood or a lone hillside, sometimes in the ditch between the properties. Between forty and fifty years ago a farmer in the parish of Keith, a tenant of the Earl of Fife, conveyed the carcase of one of his animals to a hill in the property of the Earl of Seafield.* About Pendle, Lancashire, according to Messrs. Harland and Wilkinson, when a young beast had died of the hydrocephalus, it was usual, and it has been the practice of farmers yet alive, to cut off the head and convey it to the nearest part of the adjoining county. It has been suggested that in this there is "some confused and fanciful analogy to the case of Azazel (Levit. xvi. 22), an analogy between the removal of sin and disease, that as the trangressions of the people were laid upon the head of the scape-goat, the diseases of the herd should be laid upon the head of the deceased animal." † Whether this be so or not, it seems at any rate there is the simpler meaning in the act, of intentional transfer of the disease to a neighbour's land, and this explanation seems natural enough when we consider how deep an impression the theory of transference, as we have seen, has made upon the same classes. It is true that some students of folk-lore see in transference simply a perpetuation of the scape-goat; but I cannot—when the various forms which transference presents in different parts of the world have been considered—bring myself to consider Leviticus as here sufficient and all-explaining. It may be admitted that, in course of time, what was, perhaps, the original theory of simple transference, and the more elaborate theory of symbolical or vicarious expiation, were confused or blended.

* Gregor, *Folk-Lore of North-East of Scotland*, p. 187.
† *Lancashire Folk-Lore*, p. 79.

A method of transference applicable either to man or beast was formerly practised in the north-east of Scotland. The cow, or man, diseased, was made to leap, along with a cat, through a circle made of a straw rope twisted the contrary way. The cat received the disease and, by duly dying, put an end to it. It is only one instance of the curious way in which various customs of different origin have been combined, that we have in this cure the Eastern teaching of symbolic new birth plainly indicated by the leap through the opening—a custom later touched upon—and simple transference to an animal.

CHAPTER III.

SYMPATHY AND ASSOCIATION OF IDEAS.

IN Australia, according to the accounts of some travellers, a native doctor, when his aid is sought by a sick man, fastens one end of a string to the part of the patient's body which appears to be the seat of suffering, and by sucking at the other end impresses his dupe with the belief that he is drawing forth blood, or, in other words, visibly extracting his pain. It is a simple remedy. Even more simple in its method of cure must be the copy of *The New York Commercial Advertiser* which Catlin introduced to the Minatarees, if it is still preserved. These Indians were much puzzled at the intentness with which Catlin pored over this paper. Why should he look so long at a white and black sheet? Surely it must be a medicine cloth for sore eyes. Several liberal offers were made him, Catlin says, but these he was obliged to refuse, having early in the day sold it to a young son of Esculapius, who told the traveller that if he could employ a good interpreter to explain everything in the newspaper he could travel about amongst the Minatarees, and Mandans and Sioux, and exhibit after Catlin's departure, and no doubt in course of time it would make him a great medicine man. "Just before I departed I saw him unfolding it to show to some of his friends, when he took from around it, some eight or ten folds of birch bark and deer skins, all of which were carefully enclosed in a sack made of the skin of a polecat, and undoubtedly destined to become, and to be called, his mystery or medicine bag."* Nor need we go so far afield to find instances of association of ideas operating in medical superstitions, for in the vulgar English direction to "take a hair of the dog that bit you" we have at once an example of this association, and an indication of that doctrine of sympathy which accompanies all remedies by association, except that of the rough and primitive kind given above. That dog's hair heals dog's bite has long been one of the common phrases of a village adviser, and, as I have shown in another place, within recent years the advice has been followed to apply to the wound the hair of the dog which has caused it. Dr. Dennys tells us of a distinguished sinologue who, on his missionary tours in the Canton province, was usually accompanied by a powerful dog, which, on one or two occasions, bit very slightly some of the frightened children in the villages he passed through. When a child was bitten, the mother at once ran after the dog's master to beg for a hair from the dog to apply to the part bitten.† So, too, in Madagascar the natives wear a crocodile tooth as a charm against crocodile, and so general was the dread of this animal that a golden crocodile tooth formed at one time the central ornament in the royal crown. "Man," as Mr. Tylor has said, "as yet in a low intellectual condition, having come to associate in thought those things which he found by experience to be connected in fact, proceeded erroneously to invert this action, and to conclude that association in thought must involve similar connection in reality."‡ To apply this admirable exposition to the case before us. The connection between the dog as an animal, and the bite which the dog produced, was easy to see. The dog bit, and a wound was caused. Now, reverse this.

* Catlin, *Letters and Notes on the Manners, Customs, and Condition of the North American Indian*, vol. ii. p. 92.

† Dennys, *Folk-Lore of China*, p. 52; *Folk-Lore Record*, vol. ii. "Malagasy Folk-Lore," p. 21.

‡ Tylor, *Primitive Culture*, vol. i. p. 104; see also p. 76.

The wound is here; will not the dog cure? The wound is inseparable from the bite of the dog. In one of Cervantes' novels, *La Gitanilla*, he tells of a young man, who was approaching a gipsy camp at night, being bitten by the dogs which attacked him. The old gipsy who undertook his cure took some hairs from the dogs, and, after washing the bites he had on his left leg with wine, applied the hairs, which she had fried in oil, with the oil, and covered them with a little chewed green rosemary. She then bound up the wounds with clean cloths, and made the sign of the cross over them.* That the body of a dead serpent, bruised on the wound it has caused, is thought an infallible remedy, is what one would expect.†

Dr. Dennys, when he says that a dog's virus, being powerless on its own body, a person, by swallowing one of its hairs, might hope to share the immunity enjoyed by the animal it came from, seems to me to have let the early and simple theory be obscured by the jocular meaning which now attaches to the phrase "take a hair of the dog that bit you," and to ignore what is well illustrated by the instance he gives, that originally the question was one of the assumed connection of part and whole,—in a word, of sympathy. His conjecture is, however, to some extent, supported by the direction of the leeches to administer a piece of mad dog's liver to those by whom the dog has been bitten, and by the Scotch practice of extracting the heart of a mad dog, drying it over a fire, and administering it ground to powder in a draught to the patient.‡ It is a little startling to find that in 1866, at Bradwell, a woman stated at

---

* Cited in Dyer's *English Folk-Lore*, p. 144.
† Hunt, *Romances and Drolls*, second series, p. 215. A versified proverb runs—
 "The beauteous adder hath a sting,
  Yet bears a balsam too."
From this, viper bugloss (*Echium vulgare*), from its supposed resemblance to a snake, was thought to be effectual against bites.—Annie Pratt, *Wild Flowers*, vol. i. p. 62.
‡ Dennys, *Folk-Lore of China*, p. 51.

the inquest held on the body of a child of five years of age, who had died from hydrophobia, that, at the request of the mother of the child, she had fished up the body of the dog by which the child had been bitten, and which had been drowned nine days before, in order to extract the dog's liver. A slice of this liver she cooked before the fire, and gave it to the child to eat with some bread. In spite of this treatment, however, the child died.* The reason for drowning a dog, which has bitten a person, is precautionary. The dog may not, it is true, the gossips said, be mad now, but if it should by any chance become mad hereafter, the person it had bitten would naturally, and from sympathy, instantly suffer from hydrophobia. This connection between dog and man corresponds to the connection which elsewhere was supposed to exist between the child, who had been passed through a split ash, and the tree. If it were cut down there would be little hope of the child, or man as he might then be, surviving. There does not appear to have been any reciprocal sympathy. The man might be dependant on the dog or the tree for his life, but neither tree nor dog would be affected by the death of the man arising from other causes than those with which they had to do.

It is only a step from this respect for something belonging to an animal which causes dread, as the dog among ourselves, and the crocodile in Madagascar, to a general esteem of an instrument by which a wound may have been caused. Yet the greatest teacher of sympathetic treatment, in this case, was the eminent Sir Kenelm Digby. Cornelius Agrippa, in his *Occult Philosophy*, says, " It is a wondrous thing, but easy to experience, that Pliny speaks of: ' If any person shall be sorry for any blow that he hath given another afar off or nigh at hand, if he shall presently spit into the middle of the hand with which he gave the blow, the party that was smitten shall presently be free from pain.' " " The doctrine and the employment of the ritual,"

* *Pall Mall Gazette*, October 12, 1866.

says Pettigrew, "is to be traced back to the time of Paracelsus, who, in some points of view, may be considered as the first fabricator of the powder of sympathy. Van Helmont, the panegyrist of his predecessor Paracelsus, acquaints us that the secret was first put forth by Ericcius Mehryns of Eburo," and so on, but it was Sir Kenelm Digby, without doubt, who did most for the propagation of the doctrine. Authenticity Digby guarantees to his reports by the deep study which James I. of England gave to the problem of sympathy, and James's talents and industry in matters of natural history and their origin, he says, is well known. The secret lay in its simplicity, in applying medical treatment not to the wound, but to the instrument which had inflicted the wound, or to some bandage connected with the wound. One instance will perhaps better illustrate the sympathetic theory than a page of explanation. Mr. Howell, secretary to the Duke of Buckingham, was wounded seriously in a duel; the best doctors were consulted, but in vain; even the king's own physician found the case beyond him. Four or five days after the duel, when the doctors feared gangrene would set in, and the hand be lost, the patient was in the lowest depth of misery from the excessive pain he suffered, and Sir Kenelm's advice was sought. He said he was willing to do his best, but he was, not unnaturally, afraid of being charged with witchcraft or incapacity. He was assured that the fame of his previous cures was so great that he need be under no apprehension. He then asked for a piece of cloth on which was some of the patient's blood, and he was handed part of the first bandage that had been applied. Sir Kenelm asked next for a basin of water as if he would wash his hands, and into this he put a handful of the powder he kept in the cabinet on his table, and when it was dissolved he added the piece of blood-stained cloth. After waiting anxiously for an hour he asked the patient how he felt. The reply was gratifying; he felt an agreeable coolness, he said, as if a napkin cold and wet had been laid upon his arm. Sir Kenelm assured

Howell it was the good effect of his medicine, and that if moderate heat and cold were attended to he would soon be well. The result justified his assertion. This cure was attested by the Duke of Buckingham, and James himself inquired as to the cure very narrowly, at the same time joking Digby (who hastens to remark, in a kind of literary stage whisper, that his majesty was always of most excellent amiability) on being a magician and sorcerer.

Dryden in his *Tempest* introduces this treatment. In act v. sc. 1, Ariel says, with reference to the wound received by Hippolito from Ferdinand,—

"He must be dressed again, as I have done it.
Anoint the sword which pierced him with this weapon salve, and wrap it close from air, till I have time to visit him again."

And in the next scene (sc. 2, act v.) the following dialogue ensues between Hippolito and Miranda—

HIPPOLITO: O, my wound pains me.
MIRANDA: I am come to ease you. (*She unwraps the sword.*)
HIP.: Alas! I feel the cold air come to me;
My wound shoots worse than ever. (*She wipes and anoints the sword.*)
MIRANDA: Does it still grieve you?
HIP.: Now methinks there's something
Laid just upon it.
MIRANDA: Do you find no ease?
HIP.: Yes, yes, upon the sudden, all the pain
Is leaving me. Sweet heaven, how I am eased!

The matter-of-fact explanation is, "A wound, in general terms, may be defined to be a breach in the continuity of the soft parts of the body; and an incised wound is the most simple of its kind. These, it must be remembered, were of the description of

that day in digesting, mundificating, incarnating."* So that, in fact, the beauty of Sir Kenelm's system was, that it allowed nature to interfere, far as such an intention was from the mind of either Sir Kenelm or his followers.

With the passage from Dryden that I have quoted above still in our memory, it is curious to learn from Mrs. Latham that when a man of her acquaintance fell down on a sword-stick, and cut himself severely, the sword-stick was hung at the head of his bed, and polished night and day at stated intervals by a female. We have here the Miranda and Hippolito incident, but this time in West Sussex, and in the nineteenth century. Even simple cuts are healed in the same way. The knife with which a man has cut himself should be rubbed with fat, that the healing of the cut may be hastened, and this both in England and in the Netherlands. Warenfel's note—"If the superstitious person be wounded by any chance he applies the salve not to the wound but, what is more effectual, to the weapon by which he received it,"—might, strange to say, be illustrated from many quarters. When a Northumbrian reaper is cut by his sickle he not uncommonly cleans and polishes the sickle, and from a midland county a correspondent tells me that, to cure a horse lamed by a nail, the farmers will thrust the nail into a piece of bacon, and wait for the foot to heal.

On an earlier page I have referred to that branch of association of part and whole which seeks to procure sickness or death. To bury the hair of a man, or something that had personally belonged to him, was a sure way to secure his future illness. We shall now find that exactly the same customs are followed to restore a man's health. We found, in the first instance, the enemy of a man endeavouring to bury the man's life; we now have the friend of a patient seeking to bury the patient's disease. In the county of Moray the people

* Pettigrew, *Superstitions connected with the Practice of Medicine and Surgery*, p. 163.

were formerly in the habit of paring the nails of the fingers and toes of persons suffering from hectic and consumptive diseases. The parings were put in a rag cut from the patient's clothes, and waved three times round his head, with the cry *Deas soil*. After this the rag was buried in some unknown place. Among medical men, " the Galenist of much repute," of whom Boyle writes, was induced, when other means of cure failed, to boil an egg in his own urine. The egg was afterwards buried in an ant-hill, and as the egg wasted the physician found his distemper go, and his strength to increase.* In Staffordshire, a correspondent says that to cure jaundice a bladder is often filled with the patient's urine and placed near a fire; as the water dries up the jaundice goes, and, were it necessary, many other instances of this superstition might be given. In New England, to cure a child of the rickets, a lock of its hair is buried at cross roads, and if at full moon so much the better.

A less personal connection is involved in rubbing warts with meat or snails, and then burying the meat or causing the death of the snail, but the theory of sympathy is the same. When you have rubbed the warts, a Lancashire woman will tell you, with a piece of meat stolen from a butcher's stall or basket, you must bury the meat secretly under a gateway at four lane ends, or, if you cannot conveniently and speedily find a gateway at four lane ends, you may bury the meat in any secluded spot. As the meat decays the warts go.† If the snail cure is preferred there are many ways of performing it. Some direct that for nine successive nights the snail should be rubbed on the warts and then impaled on a thorn to waste away, while others,

---

* Pettigrew, *Superstitions*, pp. 72-75 ; Boyle, *Usefulness of Experimental Philosophy*, p. 227. Pettigrew (p. 77) speaks of a similar cure of jaundice, but inaccurately calls it an instance of "transplantation." It is not transplantation, *i.e.* transference, but sympathy, and to be distinguished from the instance of transference given, *ante*, p. 35.

† Harland and Wilkinson, *Lancashire Folk-Lore*, p. 78. The practice is common in England.

and more cruelly, to cure ague, string nine or eleven snails on a thread, the patient saying, as each is threaded, " Here I leave my ague." When all are threaded they should be frizzled over a fire, and as the snails disappear so will the ague. My clerical authority for this adds, " As a note against this, I have ' from Widow K——, whose own mother was thus cured,' and I well remember how indignant the old woman was when I threw discredit upon the remedy." This was in the South of Hampshire.*

Sometimes an apple will be cut in slices, and when all the warts have been rubbed the slices will be buried ; the boy or girl rejoices that in a few days his or her warts will be gone. Or a bean-shell has been used for the same purpose, and buried secretly under an ash, with these magic words —

" As this bean-shell rots away,
So my wart shall soon decay."

In Donegal, the sufferer should seek a straw with nine knees, and cut the knots that form the joints of every one of them— any superfluous knots being thrown away,— then bury the knots in a midden or dungheap, and as the joints rot so will the warts. To cure a disease in the hoof of cattle, called " the foul," writes a Worcestershire friend, cut a sod from a spot on which the animal has been seen to tread with the bad foot, and hang it on a blackthorn bush ; as it dries the hoof heals.† If one takes as many buds from an alder bush as one has warts, and buries them, there should soon be a cure. Strike the wart downwards with the knot of a reed three times, and the same happy result will be obtained. A cure for ague, given in the *East Anglican*, is as follows:—When a fit is on, the sufferer should take a short stick and cut in it as many notches as there have been fits, including the present fit ; then tie a stone to the stick, and

* Rev. G. S. S. 16 October, 1878.
† Rev. G. S. S.; *English Folk-Lore*, p. 165 ; *Folk-Lore Record*, vol. i. p. 221; Miss E. S. 8 March, 1879.

throw stone and stick privately into a pond, which should be left without a backward look. If the strictest secrecy has been obtained, it is guaranteed by those who have tried it that the ague fits will cease. The New England practice is slightly different. First of all, the operator must learn the patient's exact name (this savours of the early disease-creating, which makes it still a matter of policy among some peoples to conceal their real names*) and the precise hours at which the chill comes on. Then send the person to cut a number of willow-rods corresponding to the time of day. Thus, if the chill comes on at ten o'clock, let him cut ten rods; take the rods one by one and lay them on the fire, saying, as each is put into the fire, "A. B. has the ague; as the rod burns, let the ague burn too," or words to that effect. When all the sticks have been burned the ague will be cured. The patient must look on in silence. The correspondent who has favoured me with this charm says, " I know a man who declares that an old woman in Canada cured him of most obstinate chills and fevers by this means, but whether every one can do it I can't say." In Sussex a snake is drawn along a man's neck if it be swollen, and afterwards the snake is put into a bottle, which is tightly corked. The bottle is buried in the ground, and, as the snake decays, the swelling goes.†

" In time of common contagion," says Sir Kenelm Digby, whose authority in matters of sympathy no student of Folk-Medicine may slight, "they use to carry about them the powder of a toad, and sometimes a living toad or spider shut up in a box; or else they carry Arsnick, or some other venomous substance, which draws unto it the contagious air, which otherwise would infect the party." The simplicity of this cure has recommended it in all cases, and although the reason given for wearing a spider or a toad is not that assigned by Sir Kenelm, we shall

---
* See *ante*, p. 20.
† *Choice Notes* (*Folk-Lore*), p. 36.

not go far wrong if we conclude that it is to the older explanation that the more modern is indebted for its origin. It will often be found that the superstitious wearer of an amulet assumes a practical and rigidly sensible position. He will not deny that he expects the odd contents of the little bag he wears round his neck to do him good. He would not wear it, he will tell you, unless he thought he had grounds, and sufficient grounds too, for believing that there is a virtue in it. Then, more probably than not, will follow an exposition of the how and the why—the ingenious exposition which has salved the half-educated man's own mind. It is by no means uninteresting, but it is generally as wide of the mark as it could well be. A glance at the charms which are in his neighbourhood, and at the nature of their composition, would do more to convince a man of the gross superstition which his conduct implies than any amount of good advice and injunctions to abjure dark practices and vague beliefs.

First, of spiders. Burton says he first saw the spider cure practised at Lindlay, in Leicestershire, by his mother in his father's house. The spider, in this instance, was put in a nutshell " lapped with silk." For long he thought this somewhat absurd, but, "at length," he tells us, " rambling amongst authors, as often I do, I found this very medicine in Dioscorides, approved by Matthiolus, repeated by Alderovandus, I began to have a better opinion of it, and to give more credit to amulets when I saw it in some parties answer to experience." Longfellow, in *Evangeline*, says :—

"Only beware of the fever, my friends ! Beware of the fever !
For it is not, like that of our cold Acadian climate,
Cured by wearing a spider hung round one's neck in a nutshell."

Alexander of Tralles speaks of tying up " the little animal that sits and weaves with the view to catch flies," in a rag, to be worn on the left arm, and endorses it as good for ague. When

Elias Ashmole was suffering from ague, on the eleventh day of May, 1681, he sought the aid of the spider. In the most matter-of-fact way he enters his treatment in his diary:—" I took, early in the morning, a good dose of elixir, and hung three spiders about my neck, and they drove my ague away. *Deo Gratias!*" The leeches directed suitable words to be said over a spider, which should be worn as a phylactery for the cure of a troublesome uvula.* " An uncle of mine," wrote a correspondent of *Notes and Queries*, " when a child, suffered from an attack of ague, and one of the medicines or antidotes prescribed for him, probably by an old nurse, was that he should wear in a bag round his neck a large live spider. He did so; but with the natural curiosity of a child the bag was opened, and upon the spider being discovered it was immediately killed. I believe the effect expected from this singular treatment was, that from the creeping of the spider in the bag, which was next the skin, a horror or disgust would be created, which would give a turn to the blood and system of the patient."† In the West of Scotland the spider was put into a goose-quill and sealed up; it was then hung round the neck of the ague patient, "so that it would be near the stomach." Sometimes more repulsively the Glasgow working-man had to make a medicine of the spider's web. One pill made of spider's web taken every morning before breakfast for three successive days was thought to bring about a speedy and satisfactory cure. This reminds us that in West Sussex many an old doctor still prescribes in bad cases of jaundice a live spider rolled up in

* Cockayne, vol. i. p. xxx. At p. 43, vol. iii. there is another spider charm. It is an incantation against a watery eruption, and was to be sung first into the left ear and then into the right, then above the man's head. " Here came entering : a spider wight : he had his hands upon his hams : he quoth that thou his hackney wert : lay thee against his neck : they began to sail off the land : as soon as they off the land came, then began they to cool : then came in a wild beast's sister : then she ended : and oaths she swore that never this could harm the sick, nor him who could get at this charm, or him who had skill to sing this charm, amen, fiat."

† *Notes and Queries*, 2nd S. vol. iii. p. 437.

butter to be swallowed as a pill, and that in New England the spider, and even a more disagreeable remedy, is administered in a spoonful of molasses.*

In Norfolk, to cure a child of whooping-cough a common house spider is tied up in a piece of muslin and pinned over the mantelpiece, and when the spider dies the cough will go.† In Worcestershire it appears that a spider in a nutshell will ward off toothache if worn in a bag round the neck.‡ The theory here seems to be that if the spider is good for one thing it should be good for another, and I do not know that any one, even now, will be able to allege a reason why it should not be as efficacious in curing toothache as in curing ague or whooping-cough.

When a Donegal peasant's child suffers from whooping-cough the anxious mother will go out in the evening, in the hope that a beetle may fly against her and be caught. When it is caught —and it must not have been looked for—the beetle is put into a bottle and carried home. As it dies the cough will go. In Lancashire a hairy caterpillar is tied round the child's neck, with the same object and the same trust.§

The instances of the use of toads or parts of toads, as Sir Kenelm Digby indicates, are also numerous. In 1822 there was a toad-doctor who travelled through the country. He cut off the hind legs of toads brought to him by his patients, and put them into small bags, which he hung round the neck of those who suffered from king's evil. The bags were to be worn until the legs inside were entirely decayed. We shall not be surprised that he travelled in his own gig when we note that for each of his bags he charged seven shillings, an entire week's wages to

---

* Napier, *Folk-Lore*, p. 95 ; *Folk-Lore Record*, vol. i. p. 45 ; Miss C. F. G. Nov. 1879.
† Dyer, *English Folk-Lore*, p. 154.
‡ Miss E. S. 8 March, 1879.
§ " Fairy Superstitions in Donegal," *University Magazine*, August, 1879, p. 219 ; *Lancashire Folk-Lore*, p. 156.

many of his patients.* The following account of a cure in the middle of the last century is quaint—"A girl at Gaddesden, having the evil in her feet from her infancy, at eleven years old lost one of her toes by it, and was so bad that she could hardly walk, therefore, was to be sent to a London hospital in a little time. But a beggar woman coming to the door, and hearing of it, said that if they would cut off the hind leg, and the foreleg on the contrary side of that, of a toad, and she wear them in a silken bag about her neck, it would certainly cure her; but it was to be observed that, on the toad's losing its legs, it was to be turned loose abroad, and as it pined, wasted and died, the distemper would likewise waste and die; which happened accordingly, for the girl was entirely cured by it, never having had the evil afterwards. Another Gaddesden girl, having the evil in her eyes, her parents dried a toad in the sun, and put it in a silken bag, which they hung on the back part of her neck, and although it was thus dried, it drawed so much as to raise little blisters, but did the girl a great deal of service, till she carelessly lost it." †

To cure fever or stop bleeding at the nose, it was thought in the south of Northamptonshire that a toad killed by transfixing it with a sharp-pointed instrument was good if the toad was hung round the neck in a bag. Dr. Jessop says that in July 1875 an intelligent grazier and horsedealer at Tintagel, who had been ill with quinsy, consulted a wise woman at Camelford. She directed him to get a live toad, fasten a string round its throat, and hang it up till the body dropped from the head. He was then to tie the string round his own neck and never take it off, night or day, till his fiftieth birthday. "You'll never have quinsy again," she said. The Wiltshire labourer wears the

* *Notes and Queries*, 5th S. vol. iv. p. 83.
† *Choice Notes* (*Folk-Lore*), p. 22, from the quaint old work by William Ellis, farmer, at Little Gaddesden, near Hempstead, Herts, published at Salisbury in 1750. Cf. Digby, *A Late Discourse touching the Cure of Wounds, &c.*, p. 77.

forelegs of a mole, and one of its hind legs, in a bag to secure his immunity from toothache.*

The right foot of a frog, wrapped in a deer's skin, is said to preserve against gout. Any one who is desirous of curing sore eyes is recommended, in Aberdeenshire, to catch a live frog and lick its eyes with his tongue. After this he has only to lick any diseased eye and a cure is effected. A cure for red water, a disease in cows, was thrusting a live frog down the animal's throat; the larger the frog the more speedy the cure.† An old woman in Donegal, who was born in the first years of this century, said, " My grandmother was that afflicted with the pains that she couldna lift her hand to her head. One day a poor woman, looking for her bit, came in an' took a seat by the fire, an' while she was there the grandmother reached up to the shelf for her knitting, an' she groaned an' lamented when she moved her arm. ' Good woman,' says the poor auld wife, ' I'm sorry to see you the way you are. What is it ails you?' Wi' that my grandmother told her all about the pains, an' she bid her get *frog's spawn* out o' the dykes, an' put it in a crock wi' a slate on the top of it, an' bury it for three months in the garden; then take it up and rub the pains wi' what she'd find in the crock. It was done, an' at the end o' the three months the crock was dug up, and the purest water was in it. I heered my mother saying that they persevered rubbing wi' the water, an' the old woman got rid of her rheumatics."‡ Helmontius praises, according to Martius, "ossiculum brachii bufonis."§ Toads made into a powder, called " Pulvis Æthiopicus," were much used internally, as well as externally, in cases of dropsy

---

* *Choice Notes*, p. 10; *Notes and Queries*, 5th S. vol. iv. p. 184; Dyer, *English Folk-Lore*, pp. 156, 175.

† Sir Thomas Browne, *Vulgar Errors*, 1658, p. 244; Gregor, *Folk-Lore of North-East of Scotland*, p. 144.

‡ "Fairy Superstitions in Donegal," *University Magazine*, August, 1879, p. 214.

§ Martius, p. 32.

and small-pox. Laid on the back of the neck alive, or dried, they were supposed to stop bleeding at the nose.*

Although, as Dalyell says, few examples are found of images formed to procure the health of a sick man, still there are some recorded. In China the figure of a man, cut in paper, is carried out into the street, in the belief of the people, *with the disease*. When the priest has squirted water from his mouth over the patient, and the paper man, and the mock money which surrounds him, the mock money and the paper figure are burned. Sprenger, when he was inquisitor, knew of a case where, when a waxen image, which had been found pierced with needles at Issbruck, was burnt, one who was sick recovered. Now, according to the general theory, the sick man should have died when his image was melted. Again, Pizzurnus is quoted to the effect that the fabrication of a waxen image has been recommended, either of the portion corresponding to a single diseased organ, or of the whole body in the case of a universal affection.†

* Bates, *Pharmacopœia;* Pettigrew, p. 783 ; Cf. Boyle, *Experimental Philosophy*, vol. i. p. 215 (quoting Henricus de Heer, *Observ. Medic. oppido. rarif.* p. 194).

† Doolittle, *Chinese*, vol. i. p. 152 ; Dalyell, *Darker Superstitions*, pp. 335, 364 ; Sprenger, *Malleus Maleficarum*, p. ii. q. i. c. 12, p. 314 ; Pizzurnus, *Enchiridion Exorcisticum*, lib. i. p. iii. c. 5, p. 54 ; " In modern India the pilgrim coming for cure will deposit in the temple the image of his diseased limb, in gold or silver or copper, according to his means," Tylor, *Primitive Culture*, vol. ii. p. 368.

CHAPTER IV.

NEW BIRTH AND SACRIFICE.

AT a period of the world's history, of which we know only that it must have been comparatively late in the history of culture, the possibility of entering life afresh—like a newly-born child—by a symbolical new birth, presented itself to mankind, worn out by struggles with invisible and visible powers, and ever-present evils of body and mind. That the old life should be left behind, with its reproaches and its regrets, that the faults and the sins of the penitent should become as it were the burdens of another, was a pleasing thing to the man who was at once weary of the old life and eager to begin a new. That the sores and diseases which afflicted the body, that the aches and pains which made day and night alike miserable, should be removed for ever, and the weak body started once again in strength and health, rose before the sufferer a tempting and fascinating dream. Whether the theory of the spiritual or the bodily new life was the first to be adopted, whether the ceremony for the latter was a copy of the former, or both were taught at one and the same time, are not only questions which show difficulties on the surface, but for the solution of which scarcely any further light is afforded us after we have considered the subject. Of the antiquity of both we can have no doubt, and that they had their origin in times prior to the Aryan dispersion would be as difficult to disprove as, I venture to think, it would be to establish.

For the spiritual new birth, as practised by the Hindus, it is directed to make an image of pure gold of the female power of nature, in the shape either of a woman or of a cow. The person to be regenerated is enclosed in, and passed through this image. As a statue of pure gold would be too expensive, it is sufficient to make an image of the sacred *yoni*, through which the person to be regenerated may go. Perforated rocks are considered as emblems of *yoni*, and through them pilgrims and others pass for the purpose of being regenerated. The utmost faith is placed in this sin-expelling transit.* It is difficult to believe that there is no connection between this ancient custom and one which prevails to the present day in Cornwall, at the "holed stone," near the village of Lanyon. Through this Mên-an-tol scrofulous children are passed naked three times, and then drawn three times on the grass, against the course of the sun. Even men and women, says Hunt, who have been afflicted with spinal diseases, or who have suffered from scrofulous taint, have been drawn through this stone, and all declare that its ancient virtues are still retained.† Many theories have been broached as to the Mên-an-tol,—that its main use was to mark the time of the summer solstice; that it is all that remains of a two-chambered dolmen;‡ that to it victims intended to be sacrificed were bound; that it was a stone of compact; but that it was a stone of healing, of transmission, seems the view taken by competent writers on the subject.§ Another hole used for the transmission of those afflicted with "a crick in the back" is the Crick Stone in Morva, Cornwall, but this stone is forked, and admittedly only a substitute for the holed stone, the higher virtues of which are conceded.‖

The most common form of transmission with the view to

* Coleman, *Hindu Mythology*, pp. 151, 175.
† Hunt, *Romances and Drolls*, first series, p. 191.
‡ *Journal of Brit. Arch. Assoc.* vol. xxxiii. art. " On some Megalithic Monuments in Western Cornwall," pp. 295, 296.
§ *Ibid.* art. " Notes on the Mên-an-tol and Chywoon Quoit, Cornwall," p. 176.
‖ Hunt, first series, pp. 191-192.

relief from sickness and disease is that mentioned by White in his *Natural History of Selborne*. In a farmyard near the middle of Selborne, he says, stood a row of pollard ashes, which by the seams and long cicatrices down their sides manifestly showed that in former times they had been cleft asunder. " These trees, when young and flexible, were severed and held open by wedges while ruptured children stripped naked were pushed through the apertures, under a persuasion that by such a process the poor babes would be cured of their infirmity. As soon as the operation was over the tree in the suffering part was plastered with loam and carefully swathed up. If the part coalesced and soldered together, as usually fell out where the feat was performed with any adroitness at all, the party was cured; but where the cleft continued to gape, the operation, it was supposed, would prove ineffectual. We have several persons now living in the village who, in their childhood, were supposed to be healed by this superstitious ceremony, derived perhaps from our Saxon ancestors, who practised it before their conversion to Christianity." * At Spitchwich, near Ashburton, in more recent days, a gamekeeper, when some remark was made on the peculiarity of an ash sapling, said that the tree had been used for the purpose of curing ruptured children. He gave details of the ceremony, and instances of the cure in the case of several well-known young men of the neighbourhood, who had been transmitted through the split in their boyhood and had grown up strong and healthy. Sometimes the patient is supposed to have thenceforth a sympathetic life with the tree; and the intelligent keeper, referring to a tree which had evidently suffered from the experiment, spoke of the deformity and sickly growth of a youth who had been passed through it.† So, too, in Corn-

* White, *Natural History of Selborne*, 1789, p. 202.
† *Reports and Trans. of Devonshire Assoc.* 1876, viii. p. 54; see also *Gentleman's Mag.* Oct. 1804; Brand, *Popular Antiquities*, p. 737; Pettigrew, *Medical Superstitions*, p. 75.

wall. In West Sussex the child, on being carried to the tree, must be attended by nine persons, each of whom passes it through the cleft from west to east.* In Germany we hear of cherry trees and oaks being used for similar purposes; thus Grimm,— "Aus dem Magdeburgischen vernahm ich folgendes: wenn zwei brüder, am besten zwillinge, einen kirschbaum in der mitte spalten und das kranke kind hindurchziehen, dann den baum wieder zubinden, so heilt das kind wie der baum heilt;" and, " In der Altmark bei Wittstock stand eine dicke krause eiche, deren äste in einander und löcher hindurch gewachsen waren: wer durch diese löcher kroch, genas von seiner krankheit, um den baum herum lagen krücken in menge die genesenden weggeworfen halten." † I do not know of children being passed through the branches of the maple for the cure of any special complaint, but in some parts of England it is thought that by so doing longevity is secured to the children.‡ In West Grinstead Park one of these trees had been long resorted to, and "when a rumour spread through the parish a few years ago that it was about to be cut down, humble petitions were presented that it might be spared." An American correspondent of *Notes and Queries*§ says that when he was a boy he saw in Burlington County, New Jersey, a tree the trunk of which had divided into two parts which met again at a short distance above. Through the opening ruptured children were passed. Unfortunately the name of the tree is not given.

Scotch witches passed children under hectic fever, and consumptive patients, thrice through a wreath of woodbine, cut during the increase of the March moon, let down over the body

---

* *Folk-Lore Record*, vol. i. p. 40.
† Grimm, *Deutsche Mythologie*, vol. ii. p. 976.
‡ *Folk-Lore Record*, vol. i. p. 43 ; also Henderson, *Folk-Lore of the Northern Counties* (1879), p. 17.
§ *Notes and Queries*, 6th S. vol. i. p. 16.

from the head to the feet.* One, more elaborately, is said to have thrown round the patient, at intervals of twenty-four hours, "Ane girth of woodbind, thrysis thre times, saying, 'I do this in name of the Father, the Sone, and the Halie Ghaist;'" and instances might be multiplied.† A good cure for any cattle disease is said to consist in making the cow, in company with a cat, leap through a loop made of a straw rope plaited contrary way and tied. The cow is cured, but the unfortunate cat dies.‡

Transmission through an artificial substance might also be effected, for the Perth Kirk Session Record of 1623 bears witness to the preparation of three cakes from nine portions of meal contributed by nine maidens and nine married women. In each cake a hole was made in order that a child might be transmitted thrice in name of the Father, the Son, and the Holy Ghost.§ A remedy quite as suggestive of new birth, though much less elaborate than this transmission, was practised near Bushire, in the Persian Gulf, for the cure of hydrophobia, some years ago. A Moollah or priest, who was a descendant of the Prophet, when consulted by persons bitten by dogs, mounted a couple of small columns of masonry a little apart from each other, placed one leg on each, and bade the afflicted pass between and under, the result being a complete cure. ‖

Again, a child in Cornwall was supposed to be overlooked ; its father and two companions burst into the witch's cottage and pinned her to the floor. The father then dragged three blazing pieces of furze from the fire and laid them across each other outside the door. He forced the child to cross the fire three

---

* Shaw, *History of the Province of Moray* (1827), p. 282, cited in Dalyell, *Darker Superstitions of Scotland*, p. 121.
† Dalyell, p. 121.
‡ Gregor, *Folk-Lore of North-East of Scotland*, p. 124.
   Dalyell, p. 394.
‖ *Notes and Queries*, 5th S. vol. xi. p. 6.

times,* thus symbolically taking her as a new being beyond the reach of the witch's power.

To crawl under a bramble which has formed a second root in the ground is said to cure rheumatism, boils, and other complaints. The arch must be complete. If it is a child suffering from whooping-cough, who is thus symbolically to be re-born, he is passed seven times from one side to the other, while the operators repeat these lines—

"In bramble, out cough,
Here I leave the whooping-cough."

"I have not a doubt," writes an Essex correspondent, "that should whooping-cough make its appearance here to-morrow, the next day the victims would be subjected to the above treatment."† In the island of Innisfallen, Killarney, is a tree called the eye of the needle. The name was given to the tree owing to its double trunk uniting. "Sure your honour will thread the eye of the needle; every one that comes to Innisfallen threads the needle," said his guide to Croker, and when he was asked what was the use of pressing through, the answer was ready, "The use, Sir! Why it will ensure your honour a long life, they say; and if your honour only was a lady in a certain way, there would be no fear of you after threading the needle." Mr Croker went through.‡

It is a fact, which could, if need were, be proved from many provincial stories, that sacrifice remains imbedded in our folk-lore. In order to avoid misconception, I should say, almost in the words of Grimm, that sacrifice has two objects and two meanings. The first object is, to propitiate those superhuman powers which have the control of health and

* Hunt, first series, pp. 236, 237.

† Hunt, second series, pp. 212, 215; Dyer, *English Folk-Lore*, p. 171; *Transactions of Devonshire Association*, 1877, vol. ix. p. 96; Rev. E. S. C. 3 November, 1879. "The newer root of such a bramble dug up, cut into nine pieces with the left hand, with ceremonies, was used to cure dysentery."—Cockayne, vol. ii. pp. 291, 293.

‡ Croker, *Legends of Killarney*, p. 46.

sickness, prosperity and misfortune; the meaning desired to be conveyed in this offering is that the favour of those powers should be continued towards the suppliant, that storms should not be sent in time of harvest, or ill-health when good health is a present possession. The second object is to conciliate the powers, should they be supposed to have exhibited displeasure—to expiate the offence which has brought about disaster,—the significance of this being, that the gods or powers are supposed to be amenable to the same influences which regulate man's relations with man. In a word, we have sacrifices to keep the powers in good humour, and sacrifices to restore good humour, for, in the dependent faith of the sacrificer, all followed in matters beyond his ken as much on the good humour of the powers as within his ken on the good humour of his fellows.

To the first class all our offerings to fairies may be said to belong. When the cream-bowl was left for the lubber-fiend, or the brownies found their wort ready, we can boldly go beyond the popular explanation that these gifts were left as rewards for undertaking that mysterious labour which the good people were credited with accomplishing in the watches of the night. It is more than doubtful if any idea of aid in return was attached to the food left in early times for the visitant. Later, when the ever-reasoning and explaining mind set itself to discover why the bowl of cream should be left, it was natural to assume that it was as a reward, or, more bluntly, a hire for work done. But in reality there was originally no idea of hire. It must be remembered that our folk-lore did not tumble down the chimney on a winter night, a complete and coherent whole. Every Jack and Jill is a descendant of a race whose origin and customs are lost in obscurity, so far as they are not shadowed forth in the daily life of Jack and Jill as we now see them, or as we may gather from what occasional scribes have told us of the more primitive ways they lived among. The bowl of cream, or whatever else was left when the household went to bed, was as much in its conception an offering to an unseen power as any sacrifice in a Pacific island. It was a petition that the powers which might come in the night should be kindly, and take of the offerings by which their servants sought to secure the continuance of their favour. This does not seem inconsistent with the later theory of hire. When the dim beings, who, although very dreadful, would share man's goods, had been forgotten as a source of possible evil, there still lingered the notion of something coming in the night. It was a natural conclusion to a practical man that if the something came and was fed, it must be because he had some reason for coming. Thus, as indicated above, the conception of hire began to dominate our tales of fairies.

To the second class belong all our medical superstitions connected with folk-lore. In Aberdeenshire, when a man is first seized with epilepsy, his clothes should be burned on the spot where he fell. This is an impromptu burnt-offering. As altars were built on places of visions or miracles, so, where the influence of the unseen made itself suddenly felt, the burnt-offering was incontinently prepared. Another cure was to bury a cock on the same sacred spot. The antiquity of the connection of the cock with sacrifice is very great. The dying utterance of Socrates was a direction to sacrifice a cock to Esculapius, to whom, with Apollo, it was dedicated. In Egypt, the red cock was sacrificed to Osiris. During the prevalence of infectious diseases in the East, Barthelemy says the cock was offered as an oblation, being sacrificed at the corners of the temples, or killed over the bed of the invalid, who was sprinkled with its blood. It is curious to note that a Scotch cure for epilepsy was to bury a cock below the patient's bed, or with parings of nails and toes, cuttings of hair, and ashes from the four corners of the hearth, at the place where the fit seized the man. Here there is real sacrifice of some portion of the man, along with the cock, in the same way that Chinese children will cut a slice off their own calves to mix with the physic ordered for a sick father's use. Five hundred years ago an Irish witch was said to have sacrificed nine red cocks to her familiar spirit, and the Buddhists of Ceylon are said still to sacrifice red cocks to evil spirits, that is, to spirits that bring evil, which must be removed. It was a red cock's blood with which Christian Levingston baked the bannock which the patient could not eat. A remedy for insanity was burying a cock between the lands of two lairds. To cure consumption Peter Levens says: "Take a brasse pot, fill it with water, set it on the fire, and put a great earthen pot within that pot, and then put in these parcels following :—Take a cock and pull him alive, then flea off his skin, then beat him in pieces, take dates a pound, and slit out the stones, and lay a layer of them in the bottom of the pot, and then lay a piece of the cock, and upon that some more of the dates, and take succory, endive, and parsley roots, and so every layer one upon another, and put in fine gold and some pearl, and cover the pot as close as may bee with coarse dow, and so let it distill a good while, and so reserve it for your use till such time as you have need thereof."*

A custom has been noticed above of hanging on a bush or tree rags that have touched a sick person, in order that a passer-by may take the rag, and with it the disease. But these rags were often left as sacrifices. Thus, when people went to St. Oswald's Well to discover by the floating or sinking of his shirt if a man would recover or not, they at their departure hung a rag of the shirt on the bush at hand. This, too, was the custom at Holywell Dale, in North Lincolnshire, at Great Cotes, at St. John's Well, Aghada, Cork, and many other places. Park, speaking of a large tree decorated with rags and scraps of cloth,

* Grimm, vol. i. p. 34 (or Stallybrass, vol. i. p. 41); Dennys, pp. 68, 69; "Romance of Chinese Social Life," *Temple Bar*, July, 1880, p. 319; Dyer, *English Folk-Lore*, p. 93 ; Dalyell, p. 86 ; Levens, 1664, *Pathway to Health*, cited in *Notes and Queries*, 1st S. vol. ii. p. 435; Mitchell, *Past in the Present*, pp. 146, 265, 274.

says that at first these scraps were probably to inform the traveller that water was near, but that the custom has been so sanctioned that nobody presumes to pass without hanging up something.* It is more conformable, however, to the rules of superstition to think that this tree served to the Africans the purpose of the votive temples of the Romans.

To avert the destruction of an entire drove it is still known that the burial of one cow alive may be useful. More cruelly, there are instances of a cow being rubbed over with tar, and driven forth from the stricken herd. The tar is set on fire, and the poor animal is allowed to run till death puts an end to its sufferings. To burn to death a pig has been recommended by a wise woman of Banffshire as a cure for cattle disease. The ashes were to be sprinkled over the byre and other farm buildings.†

Human sacrifices are, happily, now rare. Grimm says that in folk-tales there are traces of children being put to death as a cure for leprosy. Xenokrates, Galen reports, said good things of cannibalism, writing "with an air of confidence on the good effects to be obtained by eating human brains, flesh, or liver," &c.‡ Twins are regarded as of ill omen among the Barnangwato living at Shoshung in South Africa, and at the yearly sacrifice for the protection of the town from war, pestilence, or other misfortunes, twins are substituted for the orthodox black bull, and used in a decoction with which all the town is daubed.§ Tongans chop off pieces of the little finger as a sacrifice for the recovery of a relative of rank who is sick. ||

* Pettigrew, pp. 38, 39 ; *Notes and Queries*, 5th S. vol. vii. p. 37 ; vol. vi. pp. 424, 185 ; Grimm, vol. ii. p. 986.

† Lecky, *History of England in the Eighteenth Century*, vol. ii. p. 29, citing Mitchell, *Superstitions of North-West Highlands;* Gregor, p. 186.

‡ Grimm, vol. i. p. 37 (or Stallybrass, vol. i. p. 46) ; Cockayne, vol. i. p. xvii.

§ *Folk-Lore Journal*, S. Africa, vol. i. pp. 35, 36 (Rev. Roger Price on *The Ceremony of Dipheku*).

|| Tylor, *Primitive Culture*, vol. ii. pp. 363-365.

CHAPTER V.

OUR LORD AND THE SAINTS IN FOLK-MEDICINE.

IT would be wrong to charge our forefathers, and wrong to charge the peasantry of the present day, with irreverence because we frequently find the name of Our Saviour connected with trivial and apocryphal legends as to the cure of sickness. If charms were originally simply invocations or prayers, which might be of the simplest, for John MacWilliam, a Scottish wizard, simply said, "God restore you to your health," there was nothing but what was in itself praiseworthy in the mention of the name of the Great Healer. That He, in the course of His lifetime, had cured many sick and dying, the people knew from their teachers, and the natural form of any prayer on behalf of a sick daughter was, that as once upon a time Jairus's daughter was raised, so might the child of the believer; or as the woman with the issue of blood was healed for her importuning faith, so the cure of the relative on whose behalf so much prayer had been offered might be perfected. That the evil itself had been inflicted as a chastening we find acknowledged, as in the charms for the cure of sores which Lawrence Boak and his wife used, and which they acknowledged to have used when they were charged before the Kirk Session of Perth in 1631—

"Thir soirs are risen through God's wark,
And must be laid through God's help;
The mother Mary, and her dear Son,
Lay thir soirs that are begun."*

---

* *Domestic Annals of Scotland*, vol. i. p. 323.

The more general practice, however, was to couple with the name of Jesus some fact in his life with or without the attribution of a legendary incident, and then to pass on at once to an exorcision of the ailment from which the patient was suffering. For the cure of bleeding—

> "Christ was born in Bethlehem,
> Baptised in the river Jordan.
> The river stood,
> So shall thy blood.
> (*Name of person.*)
> In the name of the Father," &c.

or in prose: "Jesus that was in Bethleem born, and baptyzed was in the flumen Jordane, as stente the water at hys comyng, so stente the blood of thys man N. thy Servvaunt, thorw the vertu of thy holy name + Jesu +, and of thy Cosyn swete Sent Jon. And sey thys Charme fyve times with fyve Pater Nosters, in the worschep of the fyve woundys."

A more incomprehensible version is—

> "Christ was born in Bethlehem,
> Baptised in the river Jordan;
> There He digg'd a well,
> And turned the water against the hill,
> So shall thy blood stand still.
> In the name," &c.*

A simpler prayer, to be used in cases of nose-bleeding and wounds, given in the MS. *Liber Loci Benedicti de Whalley* (1296-1346), prays that not more "than one drop of blood" be allowed to flow. "So may it please the Son of God. So His mother Mary. In the name of the Father, stop, O blood! In the name of the Son, stop, O blood! In the name of the Holy Ghost, stop, O blood! In the name of the Holy Trinity."

When cutting the club moss (*Lycopodium inundatum*), which is good against all diseases of the eyes, the Cornish wise people

---

* Hunt, *Romances and Drolls*, second series, pp. 209-214; Brand, *Popular Antiquities*, p. 729.

first of all show the knife, with which the moss is to be cut, to the moon, and repeat—

"As Christ heal'd the issue of blood,
Do thou cut, what thou cuttest, for good."*

Sometimes the legends are difficult either to explain or trace. This may be well illustrated by the charm for toothache which is so popular among peasantry at home and abroad, and which has never, so far as I know, been explained or had its origin elucidated. One version runs—

"Christ pass'd by His brother's door,
Saw His brother lying on the floor.
What aileth thee, brother?
Pain in the teeth?
Thy teeth shall pain thee no more.
In the name," &c.

In Lancashire the following is frequently worn sewn inside the waistcoat or stays, and over the left breast:—

"Ass Sant Petter sat at the geats of Jerusalm our Blessed Lord and Sevour Jesus Crist Pased by and Sead, What Eleth thee? hee sead, Lord my teeth ecketh. Hee sead, arise and follow mee, and thy teeth shall never Eake Eney mour. Fiat + Fiat + Fiat."

Another Lancashire version, which we find amplified in Orkney, informs us that Peter "sat weeping on a marble stone," and a Devonshire charm beginning—"All glory! all glory! all glory be to the Father, and to the Son, and to the Holy Ghost!" places the scene of the incident in the garden of Gethsemane. A clergyman, writing in *Notes and Queries*, says that he once endeavoured to combat the general belief of country folks that this charm is in the Bible. He said, in

---

* *Lancashire Folk-Lore*, p. 77; Hunt, *Romances and Drolls*, second series, p. 216. "At sundown, having carefully washed the hands, the club moss is to be cut kneeling. It is to be carefully wrapped in a white cloth, and subsequently boiled in some water taken from the spring nearest to its place of growth. This may be used as a fomentation."

answer to her arguments—" Well, but dame, I think I know my Bible, and I don't find any such verse in it." But the reply was triumphant and unhesitating—" Yes, your Reverence, that is just the charm. *It's in the Bible, but you can't find it.*" In Berkshire Bortron is substituted for St. Peter.* A correspondent lately sent me a long extract from the *Inverness Courier*, which referred to this charm. A lady had tried all remedies for incessant toothache, but in vain. One of her shepherds, touched by her sufferings, asked for leave of absence, and hurried to a brother shepherd, a south-countryman, living in a glen some twenty miles off, whom he knew to have had at one time a marvellous charm in his possession. It was lent on the security of the northern shepherd's watch, and in less than half-an-hour after it had been hung round the lady's neck, her toothache vanished for ever. The charm, which was similar to those given above, was written on what seemed like an old fly-leaf, and was encased in a piece of green silk, sewn into the form of a Maltese cross. On inquiry, it was found that the charm had been introduced into the glen in the early part of this century by an Irish packman, called Ambrose Keen. " All the people about the place firmly believe that Mrs. —— was cured by the virtue inherent in this charm. As for herself, although she will not actually confess that she believes with the rest, she seems very plainly to show that she has some hidden faith in it; for I see it vexes her when any one laughs at what is a piece of superstitious nonsense."

Another legend is preserved in a familar charm against sprains and bruises. Thus, " As our Blessed Lord and Saviour Jesus Christ was riding into Jerusalem, His horse tripped and

---

* *Lancashire Folk-Lore*, p. 76 (citing Carr's *Glossary*, vol. ii. p. 264); Hunt, *Romances and Drolls*, second series, p. 215; *Choice Notes (Folk-Lore)*, pp. 62, 168; *Journal of the British Archæological Association*, vol. xxxiv. p. 329. " The belief [in West Sussex] is that the possession of a Bible or a Prayer-Book with this legend written in it is a charm against tooth-ache."— *Folk-Lore Record*, vol. i. p. 40.

sprained his leg. Our blessed Lord and Saviour blessed it, and said—
"Bone to bone, and vein to vein,
O vein turn to thy rest again.
M. N. so shall thine. In the name," &c.

or—
"Our Lord forth raide,
His foal's foot slade,
Our Lord down lighted,
His foal's foot righted.
Saying, Flesh to flesh ; blood to blood, and bane to bane.
In our Lord His Name."

The version known in Shetland is very similar, but is said in such a tone as not to be heard by the bystanders or even the person whose cure is being sought, and is preceded by the application of what is known as the " wresting thread," a thread spun from black wool with nine knots on it, to the sprained leg or arm. Grimm's remarks as to the corresponding versions in Norway and Sweden and Germany (with Oden instead of Christ) are most valuable and instructive, and to his pages I may refer those desirous of further comparing the different charms.*

The incident of the spear of Longinus is used as a charm (A.D. 1475) "to draw out Yren de Quarell":—

"Longinus Miles Ebreus percussit latus Domini nostri Jesu Christi; Sanguis exuit etiam latus; ad se traxit lancea+tetragramaton + Messyas + Sother Emanuel + Sabaoth+Adonay+ Unde sicut verba ista fuerunt verba Christi, sic exeat ferrum istud sine quarellum ab isto Christiano. Amen. And sey thys Charme five tymes in the worschip of the fyve woundys of Chryst."

Or from the *Liber Loci Benedicti de Whalley* (above quoted). " To Staunch Bleeding. A soldier of old thrust a lance into the side of the Saviour; immediately there flowed thence blood

* *Choice Notes,* p. 167 ; *Notes and Queries,* 1st S. vol. iii. p. 258; vol. iv. p. 500 ; Chambers, *Fireside Stories,* p. 37 ; Grimm, *Deutsche Mythologie,* vol. ii. pp. 1030-1031.

and water—the blood of Redemption and the water of Baptism. In the name of the Father + may the blood cease. In the name of the Son + may the blood remain. In the name of the Holy Ghost + may no more blood flow from the mouth, the vein, or the nose."

For a Stitch the leeches tell us to make a cross and sing over the place thrice,—

"Longinus miles lancea ponxit dominum et restitit sanguis et recessit dolor."*

From Cornwall we have—

"Sanguis mane in te,
Sicut Christus fuit in se,
Sanguis mane in tuâ venâ,
Sicut Christus in suâ penâ;
Sanguis mane fixus
Sicut Christus quando crucifixus."

Another from East Anglia—

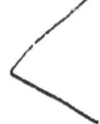
"Stand fast; lie as Christ did
When he was crucified upon the tree.
Blood remain up in the veins,
As Christ did in all his pains."

From the *History of Polperro* I take the following:—

"Christ he walketh over the land,
Carried the wild fire in his hand,
He rebuked the fire and bid it stand,
Stand wildfire, stand.
In the name," &c.†

For a Burn. "As I passed over the River Jordan I met with Christ, and He said to me, 'Woman, what aileth thee?' 'O,

---

* Brand, *Popular Antiquities*, p. 729; *Lancashire Folk-Lore*, p. 77; Cockayne, *Saxon Leechdoms*, vol. i. p. 393.

† Hunt, *Romances and Drolls*, second series, p. 214; *East Anglican*, vol. ii.; Crouch, *History of Polperro*, p. 149. Another charm is—

"Christ rode over the bridge,
Christ rode under the bridge.
Vain to vain, strain to strain,
I hope God will take it back againe."

my Lord, my flesh doth burn.' The Lord said unto me, 'Two angels cometh from the West, one for Fire, one for Frost, Out Fire and in Frost. In the name,' " &c.

The resemblance in form of this charm to that which cures toothache will be noticed, but the mention of the three angels introduces a new element. We have elsewhere three angels invoked to come from the East, " and this form of words is repeated three times to each one of nine bramble leaves immersed in spring water, making passes with the leaves from the diseased part," and a complete form in Norfolk runs as follows :—

> "An angel came from the north,
> And he brought cold and frost ;
> An angel came from the south,
> And he brought heat and fire ;
> The angel came from the north
> Put out the fire.
> In the name of the Father, and of the Son, and of the Holy Ghost."

But I have no note of any other instance in which Christ has been connected with the coming of these angels.*

Blagrave testifies that he received the following from the father of a girl who by wearing it was cured of ague, from which she had suffered two years, and also that he knew many others who had been so cured.

* Crouch, *History of Polperro;* Hunt, second series, p. 213 ; Dyer, *English Folk-Lore*, p. 169. " The child of a Devonshire labourer died from scalds caused by its turning over a saucepan. At the inquest the following strange account was given by Ann Manley, a witness :—' I am the wife of James Manley, labourer, I met Sarah Sheppard about nine o'clock on Thursday coming on the road with the child in her arms, wrapt in the tail of her frock. She said her child was scalded ; then I charmed it, as I charmed before, when a stone hopped out of the fire last Honiton fair and scalded its eye. I charmed it in the road. I charmed it by saying to myself, ' There was (*sic*) two angels come from the north, one of them brought fire, and the other frost ; out fire, in frost.' I repeat this three times. It is good for a scald. I can't say it is good for anything else. Old John Sparway told me this charm many years ago. A man may tell a woman a charm, or a woman may tell a man, but if a woman tell a woman, or a man a man, I consider it won't do any good at all.' "—*Pall Mall Gazette*, 23 November, 1868.

"When Jesus went up to the cross to be crucified the Jews asked him, saying, 'Art Thou afraid, or hast Thou the ague?' Jesus answered and said, 'I am not afraid, neither have I the ague.' All those who hear the name of Jesus about them shall not be afraid nor yet have the ague. Amen, sweet Jesus, amen, sweet Jehovah, amen."

Marsden found a similar version among the charms written on long narrow scrolls of paper, filled with scraps of verses separated by drawings, worn in Sumatra.

" + When Christ saw the cross he trembled and shaked, and they said unto him, Hast thou the ague? And he said unto them, I have neither ague nor fever; and whosoever bears these words either in writing or in mind, shall never be troubled with ague or fever. So help thy servants, O Lord, who put their trust in Thee."*

The crown of thorns is constantly introduced into rustic charms. As for the prick of a thorn—

> "Christ was of a virgin born,
> And he was prick'd by a thorn,
> And it did never bell (throb) nor swell,
> As I trust in Jesus this never will."

Or,

> "Christ was crown'd with thorns,
> The thorns did bleed but did not rot,
> No more shall thy finger.
> In the name," &c.

Or, more fully,

> "Happy man that Christ was born!
> He was crowned with a thorn;
> He was pierced through the skin,
> For to let the poison in;
> But his poor wounds, so they say,
> Closed before He passed away.
> In with healing, out with thorn,
> Happy man that Christ was born."†

---

* Brand, *Popular Antiquities*, p. 755; Marsden, *History of Sumatra*, p. 189; Pettigrew, *Medical Superstitions*, p. 57.

† Hunt, second series, p. 213; Variety in *Choice Notes* (*Folk-Lore*), p. 12; Dyer, *English Folk-Lore*, p. 173; *East Anglican*, vol. ii.; Henderson, *Folk-Lore of Northern Counties*, p. 171.

At the same time as these verses are being said, says another account, "let the middle finger of the right hand keep in motion round the thorn, and at the end of the words, three times repeated, touch it every time with the tip of your finger, and with God's blessing you will find no further trouble." Another legend speaks of the pricking with the thorn as when "Jesus walked over the earth." He pricked his foot with a thorn, "the blood sprang up to Heaven, his flesh never crankled or perished, no more wilt not thine; in the name," &c.

Agnes Sampson, the famous witch who was burned in 1590, in her exorcism of diseases, entitled "A prayer and incantation for visiting of sick folkis," conjures ills thus—

"All kindis of illis that euer may be,
In Chrystis name I conjure ye,
I conjure ye, baith mair and less,
By all the virtues of the mess,
And rycht sa, by the naillis sa,
That naillit Jesu, and na ma;
And rycht sa, by the samyn blude,
That reiket owre the ruthful rood,
Furth of the flesh and of the bane,
And in the erth, and in the stane,
I conjure ye in Goddis name."

Mother Joane of Stowe's charm for curing the diseases of beasts as well as those of men and women, as given in Lord Northampton's *Defensative against the Poyson of supposed Prophecies*,* does not differ save in a few words from those above given.

The cross itself is invoked in a curious charm, which, I was informed by the anonymous correspondent who sent me a copy, roughly printed and creased as by much folding, is still sold to Irish emigrants as they leave Queenstown.

* London, 1583, 4to.; Pettigrew, *Medical Superstitions*, p. 59.

"THE FOLLOWING PRAYER.

"The following prayer was found in the tomb of Our Lord Jesus Christ, in the year 803, and sent from the Pope to the Emperor Charles as he was going to battle for safety. They who shall repeat it every day, or hear it repeated, or keep it about them, shall never die a sudden death, nor be drowned in water, nor shall poison have any effect upon them; and it being read over any woman in labour she will be delivered safely, and be a glad mother, and when the child is born lay this on his or her right side, and he or she shall not be troubled with any misfortunes; and if you see any one in fits, lay it on his or her right side, and he or she shall stand up and thank God, and they who shall repeat it in any house shall be blest by the Lord; and he that will laugh at it will suffer. Believe this for sertain (*sic*); it is as true as if the Holy Evangelists had written it. They who keep it above them shall not fear lightning nor thunder, and they who shall repeat it every day shall have three days' warning before their death :—

THE PRAYER.

" O! adoorable (*sic*) Lord and Saviour Jesus Christ, dying on the Sacred Tree for our lives; O! Holy Cross of Christ, see me in thought; O! Holy Cross of Christ, ward off from me all sharp repenting words; O! Holy Cross of Christ, ward off from me all weapons of danger; O! Holy Cross of Christ, ward off from me all things that are evil; O! Holy Cross of Christ, protect me from my enemies; O! Holy Cross of Christ, protect me in the way of happiness; O! Holy Cross of Christ, ward off from me all dangerous deaths and give me life always; O! crucified Jesus of Nazareth, have mercy on me, now and for ever. Amen.

"In honour of our Lord Jesus Christ, and in honour of His sacred passion, and in honour of His holy resurrection, of God-like ascension, to which He liked to bring me to the right way to Heaven, true as Jesus Christ was born on Christmas Day in the stable, true as Jesus Christ was crucified on Good Friday, true as the three wise kings brought their offerings to Jesus on the third day; true as He ascended into Heaven so the honour of Jesus will keep me from my enemies, visible and invisible, now and for ever. Amen.

"O! Lord Jesus Christ, have mercy on me; Mary and Joseph, pray for me, th(r)ough Nicodemus and Joseph who took our Lord down from the Cross and buried Him. O! Lord Jesus Christ, through Thy suffering on the Cross, for truely (*sic*) your soul was parting out of this sinful world, give me grace that I may carry my cross patiently with dread and fear when I suffer, and that without complaining, and that through Thy suffering I may escape all dangers, now and for ever. Amen."

It is scarcely necessary to say that the sign of the cross occupies an important place in the prescriptions of the people. In Shropshire a cross is made on the flour after putting it to rise for baking, and also on the malt, in mashing up for brewing, to prevent each from being bewitched. To cure a sleeping foot cross it with saliva. For hiccough you may cross the front of the left shoe with the forefinger of the right hand, while you repeat the Lord's Prayer backwards.* If a man have sudden ailments, say the leech books, make three marks of Christ, one on the tongue, one on the head, and one on the breast; he will soon be well. According to the Patriarch Helias's advice to King Alfred, "Petroleum is good to drink simple for inward tenderness and to smear on outwardly on a winter's day, since it hath very much heat; hence one shall drink it in water; and it is good if for any one his speech faileth then him take it, and make the *mark of Christ* under his tongue and swallow a little of it.

---

* *Notes and Queries*, 5th S. vol. iii. p. 465; Hunt, *Romances and Drolls*, second series, p. 240; *Choice Notes* (*Folk-Lore*), p. 11; Miss E. S. 8 March, 1879. See Aubrey, *Remaines of Gentilisme*, p. 51.

Also if a man become out of his wits then him take part of it, and make Christ's mark on every limb, except the cross upon the forehead, that shall be of balsam, and the others (also) on the top of his head." Hunt says he remembers when quite a child being taken to an old woman to have a large "seedy wart" removed. Two charred sticks were taken from the fire and carefully crossed over the wart while some words were muttered. "I know not how long it was before the wart disappeared, but certainly at some time it did so." In North Hants a common charm for cramp consists in putting the shoes and stockings at bedtime in a position which somewhat resembles a cross. In Hampshire the ague patient makes three crosses, with white chalk, on the back of the kitchen chimney, that in the centre being larger than the other two, and as the fire-smoke blackens them so will the ague disappear. Hot cross buns in Tenby are hung up in a bag in the kitchen from one Good Friday to another, as a ready all-heal and medicine for man or beast.*

The association of cure of whooping-cough with rides on a donkey is due to the cross on the animal's back It is said to have been placed there, in some mysterious way, after Christ's entry into Jerusalem. The child who is suffering from whooping-cough should be placed on a donkey which has the cross on its back well defined; then, according to Dorsetshire usage, the child and donkey should be taken to where four roads meet, and ridden up and down slowly several times. The woman who told my informant declared that she had done it to all her children save one,—that one, who was too delicate to be put on the donkey at the early age customary, was the only one of a very numerous family that had the cough, and she nearly died of it. In Gloucestershire a few hairs from the donkey's cross are sewn

---

* Hunt, second series, p. 211; *Choice Notes* (*Folk-Lore*), p. 11; *Athenæum*, 11 August, 1849; Dyer, *English Folk-Lore*, p. 162; Sikes, *British Goblins*, p. 267.

up in a black silk bag, and hung round an infant's neck when teething, as this will prevent fits or convulsions.*

The apocryphal correspondence between our Lord and Abgar, King of Edessa, is frequently found in Devonshire and Shropshire cottages. It is looked upon as a genuine epistle of Christ, and as a preservative from fever. "Si quis hanc epistolam secum habuerit, securus ambulet in pace." The custom is an ancient one.†

Against all but incubi and succubi, according to Sinistrarius, the power of holy names and signs extends. "Enfin pour mettre en fuite le mauvais Démon, pour le faire trembler et frémir, il suffit, comme l'écrit Guaccius, du nom de Jésus ou de Marie, du signe de la croix, de l'approche des saintes reliques ou des objets bénits, des exorcismes, adjurations ou injonctions des prêtres; c'est ce qu'on vait tous les jours dans le cas de énergumenes, et Guaccius en rapporte maints exemples tirés des jeux nocturnes des Sorcières, où, au signe de la croix formé par l'un des assistants, au nom de Jésus simplement prononcé, Diables et Sorcières disparaissent tous ensemble. Les Incubes au contraire—."‡

* Mrs. P. 30 November, 1879; *Notes and Queries*, 5th S. vol. i. p. 204. "There were some doggerel lines connected with the ceremony, which have escaped my memory, and I have endeavoured in vain to find any one remembering them. They were to the effect that, as Christ placed the cross on the ass's back when he rode into Jerusalem, and so rendered the animal holy, if the child touched where Jesus sat it should cough no more."—Hunt, second series, pp. 218-219.

† *Notes and Queries*, 5th S. vol. i. pp. 325, 375, 376 (citing Cureton, *Ancient Syriac Documents*, 1864; Jones, *New and Full Method of Settling the Canonical Authority of the New Testament*, 1827, vol. ii. p. 2).

‡ "Ulterius malus Daemon, ut ex Peltano et Thyreo scribit Guaccius, *Compend. Malef.* lib. i. c. 19, fol. 128, ad prolationem nominis Jesu aut Mariae ad formationem signi Crucis, ad approximationem sacrarum Reliquiarum, sive rerum benedictarum, et ad exorcismos, adjurationes, aut praecepta sacerdotum, aut fugit aut pavet, concutiturque, et stridet, ut conspicitur quotidie in energumenis, et constat ex tot historiis, quas recitat Guaccius, ex quibus habetur, quod in nocturnis ludis Sagarum facto ab aliquo assistentium signo Crucis, aut pronuntiato nomine Jesu, Diaboli et secum Sagae omnes disparuerunt. Sed Incubi—," &c. *De la Démonialité*, &c. par. C. R. P. Louis Marie Sinistrari d'Ameno traduit par Isidor Liseux, pp. 128 *et seq.*

Reference will elsewhere be made to the sacrament rings made (or supposed to be made, for too often the silversmiths played the faithful a trick) of sixpences or threepences collected from nine bachelors, if the patient were a female, and from nine spinsters if the patient were a man. But this is perhaps the proper place to note that in Yorkshire in the beginning of this century, sufferers from whooping-cough would frequently resort, Protestants as well as Roman Catholics, to drink holy water out of a silver chalice,—which might not be touched by the patient,—as in Ireland weakly children are taken to drink the ablution, that is the water and wine with which the chalice is rinsed after the priest has taken the communion—the efficacy arising from the cup having just before contained the blood of our Lord. The common fame of the chalice cure for whooping-cough may be gathered from its mention in one of the *C. Mery Tales*: —" and incontynent," runs Tale xxxix. "thys gentylman went to the preest and sayd: syr, here is a skoller, a kynnysman of myne, gretly dyseasyed wyth the chyncough [whooping-cough]. I pray you, when masse is donne, gyve hym iii. draughtys of your chales. The preest grantyd hym, and tornyd hym to the skoler, and sayd: syr, I shall serue you as sone as I have sayd masse. The skoler than taryed styll and herd the mas, trusting that whan the masse was done, that the preste wold give hym hys typet of sarcenet. Thys gentylman in the mean whyle departyd out of the chyrche. Thys preste, whan mas was done, putte wyne in the chales, and cam to the skoler knelying in the pew, profferyng him to drynk of the chales. Thys skoler lokyed upon hym, and musyd and sayd: why, master parson, wherfore profer ye me the chales? Mary, quod the prest, for the gentylman told me ye were dysseasyd with the chyncough, and prayd me therfor that for a medecyne ye might drynk of the chales. Nay, by seynt mary, quod the scoler, he promysyd me ye shulde delyuer me a tipet of sarcenet. Nay, quod the preest, he spake to me of no typet, but he desyred me to gyve you drynk of the chales for the chyncough," &c.* The parish monthly nurse of Churcham, Gloucestershire, used invariably after public baptism to wash out the mouth of the infant with some of the remaining sanctified water,—it was a safeguard against toothache. Such water was so much valued for charms in Cornwall, that formerly all the fonts had to be kept locked that the people might not steal it. In the puritan west of Scotland it was looked upon as having virtue to cure many disorders—further it was a preventive against witchcraft, and eyes bathed with it would never see a ghost.† A drink of herbs (githrife, cynoglossum, yarrow, lupin, betony, &c.) worked up off clear ale was recommended for a fiend-sick patient. Seven masses were to be sung over the mixture, and garlic and holy water added. The patient should then sing the psalm Beati immaculati, and Exurgat, and Salvum me fac, deus, and drink the preparation *out of a church-bell.* The priest, when all was finished, sang over him, Domine, sancte pater omnipotens.‡ A second Confirmation is sometimes resorted to in West Sussex, in the belief that the bishop's blessing will cure any ailment from which the person may be suffering.§ To carry a child suffering from whooping-cough into three parishes, fasting, on a Sunday morning, used to be thought in Devonshire to be likely to be of great service. Other Devonshire prescriptions were: for fits, that the patient should go into a church at midnight and walk three times round the Communion table; for the cure of sore breasts, to go to church at midnight

* *Choice Notes*, p. 216; *Notes and Queries*, 1st S. vol. iii. p. 220; *A C. Mery Tales* (*Shakspere Jest-Books*), 1864, pp. 60 *et seq.*

† *Notes and Queries*, 5th S. vol. i. p. 383; Hunt, second series, p. 213; Napier, *Folk-Lore*, p. 140. To prepare a holy salve if one have not enough butter: "*Hallow some water with the hallowing of the baptismal font*, and put the butter into a jug, then take a spoon and form it into a bristle brush; write in front these holy names, Matthew, Mark, Luke, John." After singing psalms and chants a mass priest was to hallow the necessary herbs.—Cockayne, vol. iii. p. 25.

‡ Leechbook, i. ch. lxiii.; Cockayne, vol. ii. p. 139.

§ *Folk-Lore Record*, vol. i. p. 46. "I have heard of an old woman who was confirmed several times, because she thought it was good for her rheumatism."

and cut off some lead from every diamond pane in the windows, and with the lead thus obtained to make a heart to be worn by the patient.* A leaden heart was also prescribed in the North East of Scotland, but it was made thus. A sieve for sifting meal was put on the head of the patient, who was seated. In the sieve was placed, in the form of a cross, a comb and a pair of scissors, and over them a three-girded cog. Into the cog water was poured, and melted lead slowly dropped from a height into the water. The water was then carefully inspected, to see if any of the pieces of lead resembled a heart. If none of the pieces were suitable, the process was repeated until a rough heart was discovered, it was sewn up in a piece of cloth, and worn constantly by the patient. Sometimes the water and the lead were both poured through one of the loops of the scissors, and the patient either buried the heart where two lairds' lands met, or kept it under lock and key. "Ghen ony thing be oot o'ts place," said the operator during the ceremony, "may the Almichty in's mercies fesst back."†

To go fully into the cures said to have been wrought by the saints would be beyond my purpose, and would indeed require not one volume to itself but many.‡ To the honoured names of Joseph and Mary, however, English peasants still bear special reverence when they send a child suffering from whooping-cough to a house where these are the names of the master and

---

* *Notes and Queries*, 1st S. vol. ix. p. 239; *Choice Notes* (*Folk-Lore*), p. 218; *Notes and Queries*, 1st S. vol. iii. p. 258; vol. viii. p. 146; *Choice Notes* (*Folk-Lore*), pp. 168-169.

† Gregor, *Folk-Lore of North-East of Scotland*, p. 43.

‡ Among others the following saints are invoked against diseases: St. Anthony against inflammation; St. Apollonia and St. Lucy against the toothache; St. Benedict against the stone and poison; St. Blaise against bones sticking in the throat, fires, and inflammation; St. Christopher and St. Mark against sudden death; St. Clara against sore eyes; St. Genow against the gout; St. John against epilepsy and poison; St. Margaret and St. Edine against danger in child-bearing; St. Otilia against sore eyes and headache; St. Petronilla and St. Genevieve against fevers; St. Quintan against coughs; St. Ruffin against madness; St. Wolfgang against lameness.—*See* Brand, p. 197.

mistress. The child must ask, or rather demand, for there should be no courtesy prefix, bread and butter. Joseph must cut the bread, and Mary butter it and give it to the child, then a cure will certainly follow.* In the preparation of a drink for the phrensied, the Saxon leech recommended, besides recitations of litanies and the paternoster, that over the herbs twelve masses should be sung in honour of the twelve apostles.†

In the course of one of the charms given above, it will be noticed that a cure is asked, not only for our Lord's sake but for that of "Thy cousin sweet St. John." The name of St. John is indeed connected with many charms and superstitious customs. Old roots pulled from under the root of the mugwort were, according to the Practice of Paul Barbette (1675), good for cure of the falling sickness, if gathered on the eve of St. John Baptist about twelve at night, and the saint's day itself was generally devoted to the collection of herbs for secret purposes.‡ Possibly from some confusion of names the Gospel of John acquired its magical reputation. Sinistrari d'Ameno says: "à se confier en Dieu, à user frequemment de la confession; il lui persuada de lui faire sa confession sacramentelle, récita avec lui les pseaumes *Exsurgat Deus* et *Qui habitat*, et l'Evangile de Saint Jean." Auerhan, in the *Life of Wagner*, complains that the Gospel of St. John and the Psalms are wont to be used in conjurations against such spirits as himself. Valdes in *Dr. Faustus* § says—

* In Cornwall the spouses must bear the names of John and Joan. Mrs. Whitcombe, *Bygone Days in Devon and Cornwall*, p. 147, cited by Dyer, *English Folk-Lore*, p. 153. "Some deemed inscribed amulets useless unless written on virgin parchment, suspended towards the sun by three threads, which had been spun by a virgin named Mary." Martin de Arles, § 38; Dalyell, p. 390.
† Cockayne, vol. ii. p. 139.
‡ Brand, p. 183; Dalyell, *Darker Superstitions of Scotland*, p. 114.
§ *De la Démonialité*, p. 157; *Life of Wagner*, c. xxv.; *Dr. Faustus*, sc. i. lines 150-153. "The use of the first verses of the Gospel of St. John in conjurations is constantly recommended in the handbooks of magic."—Prof. Ward, note, p. 141.

"Then haste thee to some solitary grove,
And bear wise Bacon's and Albanus' works,
The Hebrew Psalter, and New Testament."

If the children of the Irish had not a piece of wolf's skin round their necks, they had the beginning of St. John's Gospel. Burton says that Jaspar Beza, a Jesuit, cured a mad woman by hanging this Gospel about her neck, and "many such," in the water. Holy water had effected cures in Japan. When the Tigretier seizes Abyssinians it causes first violent fever, and then a lingering sickness, often ending in death. The remedy generally sought is the assistance of a learned Dofléer, who reads the Gospel of St. John, and drenches the patient with cold water daily for seven days, and if he survive this he may be expected to recover. This reminds us that in the Chinese tale of the Talking Pupils, Fang is cured of blindness by a man reading the *Kuang-minrg* sutra to him.* St. John the Evangelist was said to have drunk poison without hurt, so drinks consecrated to him were believed by Teutonic tribes to prevent all danger of poisoning.†

Of the merits attributed to other saints, I can only speak briefly, for it is difficult to distinguish between genuine instances of the people's continued reliance on a particular saint and the legendary associations which give his name prominence in religious records. St. Blaze, Bishop of St. Sebaste, and martyr A.D. 288, since he restored to life a boy who had been suffocated by a fishbone, has been invoked against sore throats, and thorn pricks are also in his domain. The daughter of the Tribune Quirinus was cured of some disorder in the throat by kissing the chains of St. Peter. St. Nacaise was besought on

---

* Brand, p. 339; Burton, *Anatomy of Melancholy*, p. 298; Hecker, *Epidemics of the Middle Ages*, p. 124; Giles, *Strange Stories*, vol. i. p. 6.

† Grimm, *Deutsche Mythologie*, vol. i. p. 50 (Stallybrass, vol. i. p. 61). With John's name was associated that of Gertrude, because "Gerdrut verehrte den Johannes über alle heiligen." To their united names *minne* was drunk by friends at parting, and by travellers.

behalf of small-pox patients,--" In the name of our Lord Jesus Christ, may the Lord protect these persons, and may the work of these virgins ward off the small-pox. St. Nacaise had the small-pox, and he asked the Lord (to preserve) whoever carried his name inscribed, O, St. Nacaise! thou illustrious bishop and martyr, pray for me a sinner, and defend me by thy intercession from this disease. Amen." * We have evidently here an old legend.

St. Apollonia was the chief recognised healer of toothache, despite the incessant mention of St. Peter in charms. At her martyrdom in Alexandria, under the Emperor Philip, her teeth were beaten out. Her emblems are, " Holding a tooth in pincers. Her teeth pulled out. Pincers in left hand ; tooth in right. Pincers alone. Tied to a pillar and scourged." The Spanish legend, while resembling that of St. Peter, makes St. Apollonia suffer in heaven. "Apollonia was at the gate of heaven, and the Virgin Mary passed that way, ' Say, Apollonia, what are you about? Are you asleep or watching?' ' My lady, I neither sleep nor watch ; I am dying with a pain in my teeth.' ' By the star of Venus and the setting sun, by the most Holy Sacrament which I bore in my womb, may no pain in your teeth, neither front nor back, ever affect you from this time henceforward.' "†

St. Guthlac's belt was good against headache, and the penknife, boots, and part of the shirt of Becket were useful to aid parturition. A commemoration of St. George was thought in the Philippine Islands to protect one's rest against the scorpions.‡

* Miss Busk, *Valleys of Tirol*, p. 38 (note) ; Scot, *Discoverie of Witchcraft*, p. 137 ; Brand, p. 189 ; Pettigrew, p. 82.

† Husenbeth, *Emblems of Saints*, p. 17; *Notes and Queries*, 5th S. vol. xi. pp. 515, 516 ; " St. Appolin the rotten teeth doth keep when sore they ache ;" Barnaby Googe ; *Don Quixote*, 1842 (Jervis's translation), vol. ii. p. 73, note on the remark of the Don's housekeeper, " The orison of St. Apollonia, say you ? That might do something if my master's distemper lay in his teeth, but, alas! it lies in his brain." See also *Homily against Peril of Idolatry*.

‡ Pettigrew, pp. 42, 78.

St. Veronica's aid was invoked in Anglo-Saxon spells,[*] and St. Marchutus and St. Victricius for convulsions. Like Dr. Panegrossi, when he saw the remarkable cure effected by the Blessed John Berchmans, "When such physicians interfere, *we* have nothing more to say."[*]

[*] For the miraculous cure of the Emperor Tiberius at the sight of St. Veronica's portrait of Christ, see *Journal of the British Archæological Association*, vol. xxxvii. p. 239, art. "Apocryphal Legends."

CHAPTER VI.

CHARMS CONNECTED WITH DEATH OR THE GRAVE.

IN an earlier chapter reference has been made to the superstition which still lingers in our rural districts, that mischief can be brought upon a person enjoying good health by, in some way, bringing him into contact, with a hair it may be, of a dead man. Thus, in Devonshire, the belief was noticed that the ague can be given to a neighbour by burying such a hair under his threshold, and in New England mere walking over graves will cause incurable cramp in the foot. We have now to consider the other side of the question, to consider how disease can, according to popular belief, be cured through contact with the victims of mortality, or their relics. It would seem to be a hidden belief that life is buried with a man, and that that life can be taken, in some cases, back again, to keep those whose supply of the vital flame is small, still among the living.

In November, 1876, a correspondent of a Manchester newspaper related that he had lately been requested by a respectable tradesman to allow his man to assist in taking a young man, much afflicted with fits, to the parish church of Warningham, near Sandbach, at midnight, for if the young man could fetch a handful of earth off the grave most recently made, when the clock was striking twelve, it was believed that it would cure him. The ceremony was actually gone through, but with what results we are not informed. So, too, in Launceston, it is said that a swelling on the neck may be cured by the patient going before sunrise, on the first of May, to the grave of the last young man who has been buried, if the patient is a woman; and if a man, then to the grave of the young woman who has been last buried, and applying the dew gathered by passing the hand three times from the head to the foot of the grave, to the part affected. A similar procedure was known in Devonshire. A friend of the patient was directed to go into a churchyard on a *dark* night (the darkness was imperative), and to the grave of a person who had been interred the day previous, walk six times round the grave, and crawl across it three times. A woman had to do this if the patient was a man, and if a woman the duty devolved upon a man.*

The grass in the churchyard of St. Edrius, in South Wales, in the year 1848, was eaten by a woman bitten by a dog, for it was believed to be an antidote to hydrophobia. Henderson, quoting from the Wilkie MS., tells us that the blacksmith of Yarrowfoot's younger apprentice " was at last restored to health by eating butter made from the milk of cows fed in kirkyards, a sovereign remedy for consumption brought on through being witch-ridden." " Das grab des heiligen," Grimm says, " trägt einen birnbaum, von dessen fürchten kranke als bald genesen."†

The powder of a man's bones, burnt, and particularly that made from a skull found in the earth, was esteemed in Scotland as a cure for epilepsy. As usual, the form runs that the bones of a man will cure a woman, and the bones of a woman will cure a man. Grose notes the merits of the moss found growing upon a human skull if dried, and powdered and taken as snuff in cases of headache, and Boyle, in his essay on the *Porousness of Animal Bodies*, says, " Having been one summer frequently subject to bleed at the nose, and reduced to employ several remedies to check that distemper; that which I found the most effectual to staunch the blood was some moss off a dead man's

---

* *Choice Notes (Folk-Lore)*, p. 8 ; *Trans. Devonshire Association*, 1867, vol. ii. p. 39.

† *Maidstone Gazette*, 12 September, 1848 ; Henderson, *Folk-Lore of Northern Counties*, p. 192 ; Grimm, *Deutsche Mythologie*, vol. ii. p. 996.

skull (sent for a present out of Ireland, where it is far less rare than in most other countries), though it did but touch my skin till the herb was a little warmed by it." For fits, twenty years ago, a collier's wife applied to the sexton of Ruabon church for "ever so small a portion of human skull for the purpose of grating it similar to ginger;" she intended to add the powder to a mixture she proposed giving to her daughter. Floyer says, moss off a man's skull is like common moss, of an earthy smell, and of a rough earthy taste. He says it is much used for stopping hæmorrhages, that applied to the nose it may help the congealing of the blood, and act as an astringent, and that it may disturb the fanciful when they hold it in the hand, and by occasioning some terror may stop bleeding. Dalyell speaks of the great virtue supposed to attach to powder made from the remains of the dead, and the consequent violation of graves, and, among other cases, mentions that of John Neill, who was convicted, in March 1631, of consulting with Satan regarding the destruction of Sir George Home. First of all Neill got "fra the devill of ane inchantil dead foill" to be put in Sir George's stable "under the hek [or rack] or manger thereof: and nixt getting of ane deid hand, also inchantit be the devill, to be put in the said Sir George's yaird in Beruik, and for laying of the said foill, and deid hand in the seuerall pairtis abone writtin," but Father Arrowsmith's hand brought about notable cures in Lancashire.* A knife that has killed a man is said in China to guard from disease, and an Irish love charm was made from a strip of skin taken with a black-handled knife from a male corpse, which had been nine days buried.†

* *Domestic Annals of Scotland*, vol. iii. p. 54; Boyle, Works, vol. iv. p. 767; *Stamford Mercury*, 8 October, 1858; Floyer, *Touchstone of Medicines*, vol. i. p. 154; Dalyell, p. 380.
† Dennys, *Folk-Lore of China*, p. 51; *Irish Popular and Medical Superstitions*, p. 3. "Having restored the corpse to the grave the strip of skin is next stretched upon a tombstone, and over it certain spells are cast, and certain incantations pronounced by the attendant priestess, who sprinkles it with water found in the

In North Hants a tooth taken from the mouth of a corpse is often enveloped in a little bag, and worn round the neck to secure the wearer against toothache, but Martius says, although the friction of a dead man's tooth may be good for toothache, yet, "teste Helmontio," the loss of the patient's teeth is likely to follow.* In the north-east of Scotland the sufferer required to pull with his own teeth a tooth from the skull.

Those who steal the bones of people who have been burnt to death, or the bodies of illegitimate children, for the purpose of compounding medicines, are looked upon with such horror in China that it is said when they are born again it will be without ears, or eyes, or with hand, foot, mouth, lips or nose maimed in some way or other. It will be remembered that among the miscellaneous contents of the witches' cauldron was—

> "Finger of birth-strangled babe,
> Ditch-delivered by a drab."

John Fian, the leader of the witches and warlocks, who endeavoured by storms to prevent King James from bringing home his bride, when he visited churchyards at night to dismember bodies for his charms, preferred the bodies of unbaptised infants. No wonder Scotch parents "often on calm nights heard the wailing of the spirits of unchristened bairns among the trees and dells."†

Water found in the coffin of the Maid of Meldon in Newminster Abbey was said to be a specific in removing warts. The graves of the notable were always credited with peculiar virtues, as Grimm says: " Den gräbern der heiligen wurde in MA. unmittelbares heilvermögen beigemessen und alles was mit

hollow of a sacred stone, and then, folding it up in the form of a cross, places it over the beating heart of the credulous girl, who, under her dictation, mutters other incantations."

* Martins, *De Magica*, p. 32.

† Giles, *Strange Stories from a Chinese Studio*, vol. ii. p. 378 ; *Macbeth*, iv. i. 30; Spalding, *Elizabethan Demonology*, p. 113 ; Napier, *Folk-Lore*, p. 31.

ihnen in berührung stand gewährte hilfe, sogar der trunk des über knochen, kleider, holzsplitter und erde gegossnen wassers. Rasen und thau auf dem grab heilen. Beda erzählt von dem heiligen Oswald ; in loco, ubi pro patria dimicans a paganis interfectus est, usque hodie sanitates infirmorum et hominum et pecorum celebrari non desinunt. Unde contigit ut pulverem ipsum, ubi corpus ejus in terram corruit, multi auferentes et in aquam mittentes suis per haec infirmis multum commodi afferrent, qui videlicet mos adeo increbuit, ut paulatim ablata exinde terra fossam ad mensuram staturae verilis reddiderit; de pulvere pavimenti in quo aqua lavacri illius effusa est, multi jam sanati infirmi ; habeo quidem de ligno, in quo caput ejus occisi a paganis infixum est .... tunc benedixi acquam et astulam roboris praefati immittens obtuli aegro potandum. nec mora, melius habere coepit ;" et seq.*

In Scotland and in Ireland, in times quite recent, warts were washed with water that had accumulated in the hollows of gravestones. There is, at the time I write, in a poorhouse in Glasgow, a man to whom the water with which a corpse had been washed was administered with the view of curing him of fits.

Some Affghanistan Buddhist graves have repute for curing diseases, as that at Iohpan, near Gundamuck, where at the ziaret of Shaik Raheen Dad," by the use of prayer and at the same time circumambulating the grave and beating the limbs with a bunch of reeds, a certain cure for rheumatism, it is believed, will be found."†

Premature decease has a peculiar power of imparting lifegiving powers to inanimate objects. As Dalyell says, there seems to be "some indistinct notion of absorption of life by the instrument of death" involved in the principle.‡ Pliny

---

* Grimm, *Deutsche Mythologie*, vol. ii. p. 985. See the whole passage.
† Simpson, "Ancient Buddhist Remains in Afghanistan," *Fraser's Magazine*, new series, No. cxxii. February, 1880, pp. 197, 198.
‡ Dalyell, p. 129.

mentions that in cases of difficult parturition relief was expected from the act of throwing over the patient's house a stone or missile which had proved fatal at a single blow, or a javelin withdrawn from a body without having touched the ground.* So in China a knife that has been used to kill a fellow creature is regarded as a sovereign charm.† A halter with which one had been hanged was regarded within recent times in England as a cure for headache, if tied round the head; and the chips of a gallows worn in a bag round the neck were reputed to cure ague. Earth taken from the spot where a man had been slain was prescribed in Scotland for an ulcer or a hurt.‡ Kerchiefs dipped in King Charles's blood were found to have as much efficacy in curing the king's evil as had the living touch. Was not a girl of fourteen or fifteen years of age who lived at Deptford cured thereby in 1649? All physicians had been in vain; the girl had become quite blind, but at the touch of the handkerchief stained with the martyr's blood she at once regained her sight. Hundreds went to see this "miracle of miracles" as it was called.§ So in China after an execution, with the same faith, large pith-balls are steeped in the blood of the criminal, and sold to the people as a cure for consumption under the name of blood bread.‖ Lepers there some four years ago attacked and ate healthy men that they might drink their blood, under the belief that thus they would be cured of their disease.

The touch of the dead was, however, regarded with more universal respect. Hunt says he once saw a young woman led on to the scaffold in the Old Bailey for the purpose of having a wen touched with the hand of a man who had just been

* Pliny, *Hist. Nat.* xxviii. c. 6, 12.
† Dennys, p. 51.
‡ Dalyell, p. 126; 1616, *Rec. Ork.*
§ "A miracle of miracles wrought by the blood of Charles I. upon a mayd at Detford, four miles from London, 1649," quoted in Lecky's *England in the Eighteenth Century*, vol. i. p. 69.
‖ Dennys, p. 67.

executed;* and at Northampton formerly numbers of sufferers used to congregate round the gallows in order to receive the " dead stroke." The fee demanded for the privilege went to the hangman.†

The touch of a suicide's hand is reported to have cured a young man of Cornwall who had been afflicted with running tumours from his birth. Scot, in the *Discoverie of Witchcraft*, says, " To heal the king or queen's evil, or any other soreness of the throat, first touch the place with the hand of one that died an untimely death; otherwise let a virgin fasting lay her hand on the sore and say, 'Apollo denyeth that the heat of the plague can increase where a naked virgin quencheth it,' and spit three times upon it." In Storrington not many years ago, a young woman afflicted with a goitre was taken by her friends to the side of an open coffin that the hand of the dead should touch it twice; and another West Sussex woman who had suffered for years from an enlarged throat, when she heard that a boy had been drowned in Waltham Lock, set off there immediately, and had the part affected stroked with the dead hand nine times from east to west, and nine times from west to east.‡ If one who is suffering from any disease can attend the funeral of a suicide, and manage to throw a white handkerchief on the coffin, is a Devonshire belief that as the handkerchief decays so the disease will vanish.§

Symbolic burial was sometimes resorted to. On the border ground of Suffolk and Norfolk, to quote Mr. Dyer, a hole is dug in a meadow, and into this the little sufferer from whooping-cough is placed in a bent position, head downwards; the flag cut in making the hole is then placed over him, and there he remains till a cough is heard. It is thought that if the charm

* Hunt, *Romances and Drolls*, second series, p. 164.
† *Notes and Queries*, 1st S. vol. ii. p. 36 ; *Choice Notes* (*Folk-Lore*), p. 10.
‡ *Folk-Lore Record*, vol. i. p. 48.
§ *Notes and Queries*, 5th S. vol. i. p. 204.

be done in the evening, with only the father and the mother as witnesses, the child will soon recover.* Brand, in his *Description of Orkney*, says parents were wont to dig two adjacent graves beside a lake in the parish of Reay in Caithness, and there to lay their distempered children in the interval in order to ascertain the probability of their recovery, but a full description or further enlightenment he declined to give his readers.†

I have above noticed the "verter" water found in hollows of tombstones and rocks, and add here references to other waters useful in the cure of disease.

Speaking of the two wells at Newton, near St. Neots, Harrison says, "Never went people so fast from the church, either unto a fair or market, as they go to these wells," and naturally the reputation which such wells enjoyed has made reference to them in connection with Folk-Medicine a matter of some difficulty. It is not, therefore, necessary to attempt to enumerate the numerous wells—sanctified by the Church or the common consent of the people—which became celebrated as means of cure. Insane patients were dipped in Cornwall in St. Nun's Well; in the presbytery of Sterling they were taken to Struthill. To St. John's Well, in the parish of Wembdon, more than six hundred years ago, in the reign of Edward IV., an immense concourse resorted, who were restored to the health they sought. Those who drank of the Chader Well, in the Island of Lewis, two hundred years afterwards, made a bold experiment, for if convalescence did not immediately follow the draught, death would do so. It was kill or cure. So, too, there was a well in Dumfriesshire, the water of which if too strong for those who had been enfeebled by illness would cause death.‡

* Dyer, *English Folk-Lore*, p. 154.
† Brand, *Description of Orkney*, p. 154.
‡ Harrison, *Description of England* (N. Shak. Soc. ed.), bk. ii. ch. xxiii. p. 350; Hunt, second series, p. 51; Collinson, *History of Somerset*, vol. iii. p. 104; Dalyell, *Darker Superstitions of Scotland*, pp. 82, 83, 84.

Probably the best known of these wells in the present day is that of Holywell. When St. Winifred's head, as the legend goes, was struck off by Prince Caradoc, it rolled into the church of St. Beuno, the uncle of the pious maiden, and where it rested a wonderful spring came forth. The approach to the vault is by stairs, trodden in their time by many feet, but the vault itself is not inviting, nay, even depressing; the carvings are chipped and broken, and one cannot but think that the visitors of to-day are neither so anxious nor so reverent as those who of old for hours were to be seen up to their chins in the water, praying devoutly. One noble knight prolonged too greatly his devotions, for, " having continued so long mumbling his paternosters and *Sancta Winifreda ora pro me*, the cold struck into his body, and after his coming forth of that well he never spoke more." Hither came William the Conqueror, his grandson Henry II., and the first Edward; here, too, many of the Gunpowder Plot Conspirators, and later James II. The Duke of Westminster, in 1876, leased the well to the Corporation of Holywell for a thousand years at a sovereign a year. The flow is always at the same rate, and although the water is extremely cold it never freezes. At the date of a recent visit, the following left by patients, who had gone away cured, might have been seen by the curious:—Thirty-nine crutches, six hand-sticks, a hand-hearse, and a pair of boots.

When a friend was about to take water from the Dow Loch, in Dumfriesshire, it appears from an old trial that each time the vessel was raised from the surface these words were to be pronounced, "' I lift this watter in name of the Father, Sone, and Holy Gaist, to do guid for thair helth for quhom it is liftit,' quhilk wordis sould be repeitit thryse nyne times."*

The Borgie well, at Cambuslang, near Glasgow, is credited with making mad those who drink from it; according to the local rhyme—

* Trial of Bartie Paterson, 18 Dec. 1607; *Rec. Just.;* Dalyell, p. 84.

"A drink of the Borgie, a bite of the weed,
Sets a' the Cam'slang folk wrang in the head."

The weed is the weedy fungi. The story, however, must be an implied satire on the Cambuslang people generally, for the original Borgie's well, which was blocked up some years ago, was the principal water supply of the district.

To the wells of St. Elian, St. Cynhafal, St. Barruc, and others, in which patients were accustomed to drop pins, I shall elsewhere refer. It is believed that on the twenty-sixth day of June, in each year, the waters on Saw Beach, Maine, become gifted with power to heal and strengthen. People flock to the beach from all the country round for a healing dip.*

Many persons and cattle were cured by washings from a stone called St. Convall's Chariot—the stone, according to tradition, upon which St. Convall had been borne from Ireland to the banks of the Clyde. From a letter of 1710 it appears that when stones were washed the first water was poured out, and that only to the second water belonged the virtue.†

The Chinese do not approve of running water near their dwelling-houses because they say it runs away with their luck.‡ The English and Scotch peasant, on the other hand, attaches a special value to a stream because it will bear away all the evil which may beset a household. For thrush the wise woman would tell the child's mother to take three rushes from a running stream and pass them separately through the mouth of the infant, then throw them into the stream, for as the rushes were borne away by the current so the thrush was borne from the

---

* Miss C. F. G. 23 March, 1880.
† Dalyell, pp. 152, 511.
‡ "I myself knew a case of a man, provided with a pretty little house, rent free, alongside of which ran a mountain rill, who left the place and paid for lodgings out of his own pocket, rather than live so close to a stream which he averred carried all his good luck away. Yet this man was a fair scholar and a graduate to boot."—Giles, *Strange Stories from a Chinese Studio*, vol. ii. p. 110.

child.* To cure inflammation, the leeches ordered the friend of the patient to take a hazel, or an elder stick, or spoon, and cut his name thereon, " cut three scores on the place, fill the name with the blood, throw it over thy shoulder, or between thy thighs into running water, and stand over the man." So, also, the blood taken from a scarified neck, after the setting of the sun, to remove blotches was thrown into running water. When a holy drink against elfin tricks and temptations of the devil was to be prepared, it was half a sextarius of running water that the immaculate person was to bring in silence to receive the herb crystallium, and tansy, and zedoary, and cassuck, and fennel, and to wash the texts and psalms from the dish on which they had been written into the dish " very clean," which when hallowed by holy wine was to be taken to church, and have masses sung over it, " one Omnibus sanctis, another Contra tribulationem, a third of St. Mary ;" and the psalms, Miserere mei, dominus, Deus in nomine tuo, Deus misereatur nobis, Domine Deus, Inclina domine, and the Credo, the Gloria in excelsis domino," and some litanies.† Within the last few years a lady sketching on the bank of the Lennan, a trout stream not far from Letter Kenny, saw a young girl come down a sloping field on the opposite side, leading a boy with a halter round his neck. When the pair reached the river the boy went down on his hands and knees, and so led by the girl crossed the river, bending his lips to drink. They then recrossed in the same fashion; he drank as before, and she led. Then they went up the hill home. But presently they again appeared, coming down the hill. This time, however, the boy led the girl, otherwise the ceremony was in every respect the same. " Me and Tom's very bad with the

---

* *Notes and Queries*, 1st S. vol. viii. p. 265. Another version mentions only one straw, but says, " repeat the verse, ' Out of the mouths of babes and sucklings,' " &c.—*English Folk-Lore*, p. 150.

† Cockayne, vol. ii. pp. 105, 77 ; vol. iii. p. 13. Another version of the last charming will be found in vol. ii. p. 137.

mumps," explained the little girl, raising her hands to her swollen neck and cheeks, " so I put the branks on Tom an' took him to the water, an' then he put them on me. We be to do that three times, an' its allowed it be a cure." And a cure did result.* Is this superstition, the crossing the hill being borne in mind, connected with a New England superstition with which a correspondent has favoured me, that if any one living on one side of a hill or mountain suffers from sore throat, water must be brought from a well or spring on the other side, and the patient drink the water after bathing the part affected?

Water taken by a maiden for nine days from a stream which ran directly east was recommended as a cure for " ivens at the heart," but in general that the direction of the water should be from north or south was regarded as far more auspicious. Patients were instructed to wash themselves three nights in a south-running stream, and persons suffering from witchcraft were bid to do the same thing. According to the *Perth Kirk Session Record* of May 1623, the " rippillis " was cured by hog's lard, and ablution in such esteemed water. John Brough was accused twenty years later of mysteriously curing cattle and women by washing their feet in south-running water with other ceremonies. When John Neill cured George Reule he ordered Reule's wife to wash his shirt in south-running water and put it wet on the patient; and Jonet Stewart, when she went to see Bessie Inglis, " tuke off hir sark and hir mutche, and waischit thame in south-rynnand water, and pat the sark wat upon hir at midnycht, and said thrysis over, 'In the name of the Fader, the Sone, and Holy Gaist,' and fyret the water and brunt stray at ilk nwke of the bed." To cure whooping-cough in Northumberland a fire was made on a girdle held over a south-running stream and porridge cooked thereon. When this was done, not very long ago, the number of candidates, Mr. Henderson says, was so great that each patient got

* " Fairy Superstitions in Donegal," *Univ. Mag.* Aug. 1879, p. 219.

but one spoonful as a dose. A holy well in Ireland, round which the whole night a circle of pilgrims sat on May-eve, was said to be a south-running spring of common water.* According to the "Exmoor scolding," sciatica, known in the neighbourhood of Exmoor as "boneshave" may be cured by the patient lying on his back by the side of a river or brook with a stick between him and the water, while one repeats over him—

> "Boneshave right,
> Boneshave straight,
> As the water runs by the stave,
> Good for boneshave." †

---

* Dalyell, pp. 84 *et seq.*; *Witches of Renfrewshire*, p. 22 (Mackenzie, § x.); Henderson, *Folk-Lore of the Northern Counties*, p. 141 ; Richardson, *Folly of Pilgrimages in Ireland*, 1727, p. 65.

† Pettigrew, p. 64.

CHAPTER VII.

COLOUR.

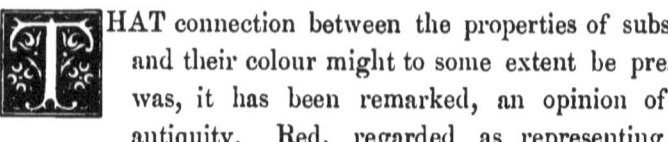HAT connection between the properties of substances and their colour might to some extent be presumed was, it has been remarked, an opinion of great antiquity. Red, regarded as representing heat, was therefore itself in a manner heat; white, representing cold, was therefore cold in itself. The superstition will be found to be very general. Red flowers were given for disorders of the blood, and yellow for those of the liver.* The flowers of the amaranthus dried, and beaten into powder, Culpepper says, stop a certain complaint, " and so do almost all other things ; and by the icon or image of every herb the ancients at first found out their virtues." " Modern writers," he continues, " laugh at them for it ; but I wonder, in my heart, how the virtues of herbs came at first to be known if not by their signatures."† " We find," Pettigrew—who accumulated some curious historical information on this point—writes, " that in small-pox red bed-coverings were employed with the view of bringing the pustules to the surface of the body." The bed-furniture, John of Gaddesden directed, when the son of Edward II. was sick of the small-pox, should be red ; and so successful, apparently, was his mode of treatment, that the

---
* Cf. " Pari quoque ratione herbarum succos, qui succos sive humores humani corporis colore referebant, in illius humoris peccantis purgationem adhibebant. Hinc croceis plantarum liquoribus bilem flavam, atris, purpurascentibus aut coeruleis nigram, albis pituitum, rubris sanguinem, lactescentibus lac et sperma valebant curare."—Heucherus et Fabricius, *De Vegetalibus Magicis*, Wittenberg, 1700.

† *English Physician Enlarged*, p. 13.

prince completely recovered, and bore no mark of his dangerous illness. So, at the close of the last century, the Emperor Francis I., when suffering from the same disease, was rolled up in a scarlet cloth. But this case was not attended with so much success, for the emperor died. A Japanese authority testifies to the children of the royal house, when they were attacked by small-pox, being laid in chambers where bed and walls were alike covered with red, and all who approached were clothed in scarlet.*

If red colours were useful in cases of sickness, one reason probably was, because they were obnoxious to evil spirits. To the present day, in China, red cloth is worn in the pockets, and red silk braided in the hair of children; and of a written charm Dennys says—" The charm here given was written on red paper, that colour being supposed to be peculiarly obnoxious to evil spirits." Red pills were administered by Chiao-no, in a Chinese tale; in one case, to cure a wound, the pill was passed round and round the place, and in another, to restore life, it was put into the man's mouth, "and presently there was a gurgle in his throat and he came round."† It was because evil spirits would be frightened, probably, that red was used so liberally at the death of a New Zealander. His house was painted red; wherever *tapu* was laid a post was erected and painted red; at whatever spot the corpse might rest a stone, or rock, or tree at hand was painted red; and if the corpse was conveyed by water, when it had been taken ashore at its destination it was painted red before it was abandoned. "When the *hahunga* took place, the scraped bones of the chief thus ornamented, and wrapped in a red-stained mat, were deposited in a box or bowl smeared with the sacred colour, and placed

---

* Pettigrew, *Superstitions connected with the History and Practice of Medicine and Surgery*, pp. 18-19.

† Dennys, *Folk-Lore of China*, p. 54; Giles, *Strange Stories from a Chinese Studio*, vol. i. pp. 40, 44, 45.

in a painted tomb. Near his final resting-place a lofty and elaborately carved monument was erected to his memory; this was called the *tiki*, which was also thus coloured."* The guardians of the ryot's fields in Southern India—the four or five standing stones—are daubed with red paint,† and Shashti's proper image is a rough stone smeared with the same colour.‡

Red was also, we learn from Merolla, a sacred colour in Congo. When a Mahometan of sanctity dies, over his grave is placed a heap of large stones, or of mud, and in the centre is a pole with a piece of white or red cloth on the end, "as a banner or signal to all who pass that a holy man is buried there, and the spot becomes famous as a resort for prayer."§ It would seem, from a passage quoted by Dalyell, that red played an important part in the symbolical destruction of an enemy in India, and it is curious, in this connection, to note that the ghosts of suicides are distinguished in China by wearing red silk handkerchiefs. When the corpse candles in Wales burn white the doomed person is a woman, but if the flame be red then it is a man.‖

It is not surprising, therefore, to find that red cords and red bands should play an important part in Folk-Medicine. In the West Indies a little bit of scarlet cloth, however narrow a strip, worn round the neck, will keep off the whooping-cough. Many centuries earlier, for lunacy one was told by the leeches

* Taylor, *New Zealand and the New Zealanders*, p. 95; Lubbock, *Origin of Civilisation*, p. 306.

† To give them eyes to watch? In China "on a certain day after the death of a parent the surviving head of the family proceeds with much solemnity to dab a spot of ink upon the memorial tablet of the deceased. *This is believed to give to the departed spirit the power of remaining near to, and watching over the fortunes of, those left behind.*"—Giles, vol. ii. p. 224 (foot note).

‡ Tylor, *Primitive Culture*, vol. ii. p. 150.

§ Pinkerton, vol. xvi. p. 273; Simpson, "Ancient Buddhist Remains in Afghanistan," *Fraser's Magazine*, new series, vol. cxxii. February 1880, p. 197.

‖ Dalyell, *Darker Superstitions of Scotland*, p. 365; Dennys, p. 75; Sikes, *British Goblins*, p. 239.

to take of the clove wort (*Ranunculus acris*) "and wreathe it with a red thread about the man's swere (neck) when the moon is on the wane in the month which is called April; soon he will be healed." In the west of Scotland it is, or was, common to wrap a piece of red flannel round the neck of a child in order to ward off whooping-cough. The virtue, our authority is careful to inform us, " lay not in the flannel but in the red colour. Red was a colour symbolical of triumph and victory over all enemies."· Is this a recollection of the red beard of Thôrr, invoked by men in distress ? *

To prevent nose-bleeding people are told to this day to wear a skein of scarlet silk thread round the neck, tied with nine knots down the front; if the patient is a man, the silk being put on and the knots tied by a woman ; and if the patient is a woman, then these good services being rendered by a man. Sore throats were cured in ancient England by wearing a charm tied about the neck in a red rag. We have evidence of the recent use of scarlet, with a sympathetic purpose, in the testimony of a correspondent of *Notes and Queries*, who writes—" When I was a pupil at St. Bartholomew's, forty years ago, one of our lecturers used to say that within a recent period there were exposed for sale in a shop in Fleet Street red tongues—*i.e.*, tongues of red cloth—to tie round the throats of patients suffering from scarlet fever." A shrewmouse, wrapped in clay or a red rag, and waybroad "delved up without iron ere the rising of the sun," bound with crosswort in a red fillet round the head, were Saxon remedies.† Salmuth mentions the use of red coral beaten up with oak leaves in the transference of an ailment. Even the jasper owes its high reputation for stopping hæmor-

* Branch, *Contemporary Review*, October, 1875 ; Cockayne, *Saxon Leechdoms*, vol. i. p. 101 ; Napier, *Folk-Lore*, p. 96 ; Cf. Giles, vol. i. p. 324 ; Grimm, *Deutsche Mythologie*, vol. i. p. 147 (Stallybrass, vol. i. p. 177). "A common mode of making up peace in China is to send the aggrieved party an olive and a piece of *red* paper in token that peace is restored." Man in the Moon ties together with a *red* cord the feet of those destined to be man and wife.—*Ibid.* pp. 121, 141.

† *Notes and Queries*, 5th S. vol. xi. p. 166 ; Cockayne, vol. i. xxxi.-ii. 307.

rhage to its blood-red colour, and Boetius de Boot relates a marvellous story thereanent.*

In Guinea the fetish woman orders a white cock to be killed when she is consulted about a man's disease, but the Buddhists of Ceylon, like the Irish of the fourteenth century, are said to sacrifice *red* cocks. So, too, did Christian Levingston by Christian Saidler's counsel, "get a reid (red) cock, quhilk scho slew, and tuke the blude of it, and scho bake a bannock theirof with floure, and gaif the said Andro to eit of it, quhilk he could not prief." †

The virtues of the sanguine colour even applied to animals; for in Aberdeenshire it is a common practice with the housewife to tie a piece of *red* worsted thread round the cows' tails before turning them out for the first time in the season to grass. It secured the cattle from the evil eye, elf shots, and other dangers. Further afield, in Carinthia, we find, possibly because, as Mr. Kelly says, "red thread is typical of lightning," that a red cloth is laid upon the churn when it is in use, to prevent the milk from being bewitched and yielding no butter.‡

It is to *blue* that we should have expected to find the most power attributed. It is the sky colour and the Druid's sacred colour. In Christianity it is the colour of the Virgin, and therefore holy; and yet it is remarkable that the mention of it in connection with Folk-Medicine is scanty.

In 1635 a man in the Orkney Islands was, we are led to believe, utterly ruined by nine knots cast on a *blue* thread and given to his sister. We can understand this, for if a colour possessed mysterious properties it was quite as certain that they

---

* Pettigrew, p. 77; *De Lapid. et Rem.* lib. ii. cap. 102, quoted by Pettigrew, p. 82.

† Tylor, *Primitive Culture,* vol. ii. p. 123; Croker, *Researches in the South of Ireland;* Dalyell, p. 86.

‡ *Choice Notes* (*Folk-Lore*), p. 24; Kelly, *Indo-European Tradition and Folk-Lore,* p. 147; Cf. Grimm, *Deutsche Mythologie,* vol. i. p. 148.

would be used if possible for hurt as for healing. On the banks of the Ale and the Teviot, however, the women have still a custom of wearing round their necks blue woollen threads or cords till they wean their children, doing this for the purpose of averting ephemeral fevers. These cords are handed down from mother to daughter, and esteemed in proportion to their antiquity.* Probably these threads had originally received some blessing. This we should suppose to have been the thread of proper colour to receive such a blessing—for, was not blue the Virgin's colour? We have, therefore, here, two illustrations of the current of the people's thoughts. In the Orkneys, the blue thread was used for an evil purpose because such a colour savoured of "Popery" and priests; in the northern counties it was used because a remembrance of its once pre-eminent value still survived in the minds of those who wore it, unconsciously, though still actively, influencing their thoughts. In, perhaps, the same way we respect the virtue of the red threads, because, as Conway puts it, "red is sacred in one direction as symbolising the blood of Christ"; and again, as in Shropshire, refuse to allow a red-haired man to be first-foot on New Year's Day, "or there'll be a death in it afore the year's out," because red again is "the colour of Judas who betrayed that blood."†

Flannel dyed nine times in blue was supposed to be useful in removing glandular swellings, but, again, the nip which the devil gave a witch, and by which devil's mark she was to be recognised, was blue. More, when the devil appeared to those forming the clay image which was to take away the life of Sir George Maxwell of Pollok in 1677, it was noticed that "his apparel was black, and that he had a bluish band and handcuffs." In German folk-

* *Rec. Ork.* p. 97, quoted in Dalyell, p. 307; Henderson, *Folk-Lore of the Northern Counties*, p. 20.
† Conway, *Demonology and Devil Lore*, vol. ii. p. 284; *N. and Q.* 5th S. vol. iii. p. 465.

lore the lightning is represented as blue, as Grimm shows quoting from a Prussian tale, "der mit der *blauen peitsche* verfolght den teufel," *i.e.* the giants. The blue flame was held especially sacred on this account, the North Frisians swearing "*donners blöskên* help!" and Schärtlin's curse was "blau feuer!" *

Eily McGarvey, a Donegal wise women, employs a *green* thread in her work. She measures her patients three times round the waist with a ribbon, to the outer edge of which is fastened a green thread. " If her patient is mistaken in supposing himself to be afflicted with heart fever, this green thread will remain in its place; but should he really have the disorder, it will be found that the thread has left the edge of the ribbon, and lies curled up in the centre. At the third measuring Eily prays for a blessing, in the name of the Father, of the Son, and of the Holy Ghost. She next hands the patient nine leaves of 'heart fever grass,' or dandelion, gathered by herself, directing him to eat three leaves on successive mornings." Generally, green is regarded as unlucky, and specially so by the Sinclairs of Caithness. " They were dressed in green, and they crossed the Ord upon a Monday in their way to Flodden Field, where they fought and fell in the service of their country, almost without leaving a representative of their name behind them. The day and the dress are accordingly regarded as inauspicious." " Green's forsaken and yellow's foresworn " is a common saying, "and blue is the colour that must be worn." Green stockings were sent to any elder sister in Scotland if a younger sister was married before her, that she might wear them as a forsaken maiden at the dance which followed the wedding, but for bridal bed-colours blue, as representing constancy, and green as repre-

---

* Pettigrew, p. 19; Sir George Mackenzie, *Laws and Customs of Scotland in Matters Criminal*, 1678; *Renfrewshire Witches*, p. 48; Grimm, *Deutsche Mythologie*, vol. i. p. 148; " Blue Clue in Hallow'een Divination," Brand, *Popular Antiquities*, p. 209 (foot-note). *Folk-Lore Record*, vol. ii. p. 204.

senting youth, were chosen, for " combine the two and you have youthful constancy." *

Turning to *yellow*, we find that charms yellow or written on yellow paper are quite as numerous in China as those written on red, for yellow is the imperial colour, one of the five recognised in the Chinese cosmogony, and a peculiar virtue therefore attaches to it. Martius says that some hang a live beetle sewed up in a yellow linen bag round the neck, like an amulet. Bridal-garters should be yellow, " signifying honour and joy." " The demon of jaundice," says Conway, " is generally when exorcised consigned to yellow parrots, and inflammation to red or scarlet weeds."†

For illustration of the use of black and white in folk-medicine we can go back to the Assyrians.

    1. Take a white cloth. In it place the mamit,
    2. In the sick man's right hand ;
    3. And take a black cloth,
    4. Wrap it round his left hand.
    5. Then all the evil spirits
    6. And the sins which he has committed
    7. Shall quit their hold of him
    8. And shall never return.

This has been explained thus—by the black cloth in the left hand he repudiates all his former evil deeds, and he symbolises his trust in holiness by the white cloth in the right hand.‡ In Scotland, in November 1596, Christian Stewart was burned as a witch, having been found " art and part of bewitching Patrick

---

* " Fairy Superstitions in Donegal," *University Magazine*, August, 1879, p. 217 ; Brand, pp. 320, 360. Cf. " Green, indeed, is the colour of Lovers," *Love's Labour's Lost*, act i. 2 ; *Antiquary*, vol. iii. p. 111 ; Gregor, *Folk-Lore of North-East of Scotland*, p. 87.

† Dennys, p. 54 ; Martius, p. 31; Brand, p. 362; Conway, vol. i. p. 284. " In certain cases a charm in China is written upon two pieces of yellow paper with a new vermilion pencil. One piece is burned and the ashes swallowed, the other is placed above the patient's door."—*Credulities Past and Present*, p. 180.

‡ *Records of the Past*, vol. iii. p. 140.

Ruthven by laying on him a heavy sickness with a *black* clout, which she herself had confessed before several ministers, notaries, and others at divers times."

In ancient Germany white sacrifices were generally considered the most acceptable, but the water spirit demanded a black lamb, and a black lamb and a black cat were offered to the huldres. Caldcleugh testifies to the blood of a black lamb being administered for erysipelas in South America.*

In England the black cat was the chosen familiar of the witches, and on this account figures so prominently in all modern tales of darkness. In North Hants to cure a stye in the eye you are told to pluck one hair from the tail of a black cat on the first night of the new moon, and rub it nine times over the stye. Blood of a black cat taken from the tail was frequently used by old women for shingles (*herpes*). It was smeared over the place affected.† I have heard of this being recommended in Ireland in recent times, but it caused, in an authentic case, considerable mischief. A three-coloured cat is said to be a protection against fire, but a black cat is credited in rather a vague way with curing epilepsy and protecting gardens. In New England the skin of a black cat is considered a remedy in cases of sore throat, and it is lucky if a black cat come to you, but to sail with one on board is unlucky; however, if the cat be killed certain ruin will follow. In the northeast of Scotland it is considered unlucky to meet a black cat at any time.‡

One Gerner, according to the Kirk Session Record of St. Cuthbert's, gave "drinkes of black henis aiges and aquavite to

* Grimm, vol. i. p. 44 (Stallybrass, vol. i. p. 54); Caldcleugh, *Travels*, vol. ii. p. 212.

† Turner, *Diseases of the Skin*, p. 79.

‡ Gregor, p. 124. Burial of a black cat's head, see Aubrey's *Remains of Gentilisme* (Folk-Lore Society), p. 102. The connection between cats and witches is illustrated in Grimm, "Das Volk sagt: eine zwanzigjährige Katze werde zur Hexe, eine hundertjährige Hexe wieder zur Katze," vol. ii. pp. 918-919.

sundrie persones that had the hert aikandes." If you have called up the devil by repeating the Lord's Prayer backwards, the only way to appease him, they say in Weardale, Durham, is to present him with a black hen.* It was by the baptism of a black cat that the Scotch witches raised the dreadful storm which assailed James VI. on his way to his kingdom with his bride.†

A cake made of the heart of a white hound baked with meal was recommended for convulsions; but to meet a white horse without spitting at it (spitting averts all evil consequences) is considered very unlucky in the Midland Counties, and to see a white mouse run across a room is a sure sign of approaching mortality to Northamptonshire people.

Agrimony and black sheep's grease were employed in combination, and for "dint of an ill wind" (Perth Kirk Session Record, 1623) black wool and butter were prescribed, probably for unction, and black wool, olive oil, and eggs for a cold. Dalyell, who notes these remedies, mentions that when he was recovering from a dangerous fever in the spring of 1826, an estimable relative presented him with some black wool to put into his ears, as a preservative from deafness. He availed himself eagerly of the gift, but declares that he would abstain from proclaiming its efficacy. The intention here was kindly enough, and if the remedy was not successful we must remember—

> Seven times tried that judgment is
> That did *never* choose amiss.

---

* The blood of a perfectly black hen will cure rheumatism, shingles, or, in fact, anything if applied externally, say some New England wise-men.

† Dalyell, p. 116 ; *Folk-Lore Record*, vol. ii. p. 205.

CHAPTER VIII.

1. NUMBER.

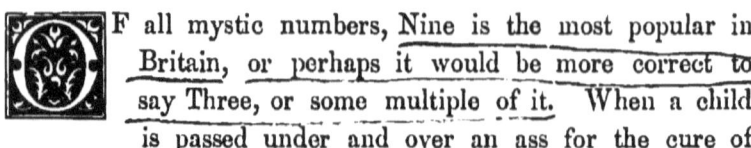F all mystic numbers, Nine is the most popular in Britain, or perhaps it would be more correct to say Three, or some multiple of it. When a child is passed under and over an ass for the cure of whooping-cough, it is always three or nine times that the operation is performed. In an Irish case the child was passed three times under and over for nine successive mornings. The Cornwall system is even more elaborate—the child is passed nine times under and over a donkey three years old. Then three spoonfuls of milk are drawn from the teats of the animal, and three hairs cut from the back, and three hairs cut from the belly placed in it. After the milk has stood for three hours it should be drunk by the child in three doses, the whole ceremony being repeated three successive mornings.* When Margaret Sandieson went to cure Margaret Mure, she took but "thrie small stones and twiched her head thrie tymes with everie one of them," which cured her speedily. From the record in the trial of Bartie Paterson, in 1607, it appears that among other remedies for an unknown disease the patient was directed to kneel by his bedside "thrie severall nichtes, and everie nicht, thryse nyne tymes, to ask his helth at all leving wichtis above and vnder the earth in the name of Jesus;" and again, he was "to tak nyne pickellis of quheit [? wheat] and nyne pickellis of rowne trie,

---

* *Lancashire Folk-Lore*, vol. i. p. 157; W. II. P. (Belfast), 26th Nov. 1878; *N. and Q.* 5th S. vol. x. p. 126; *Manchester Guardian*, August, 1876; Hunt, *Romances and Drolls*, second series, p. 218; Cf. Gregor, *Folk-Lore of North-East of Scotland*, p. 132.

and to weir thame continuallie vpone for his helth."* In North Berwick a draught, repeated nine times, from the ham of a living ox was prescribed, Dalyell says, "for whooping-cough"; together with putting the patient " nyne severall tymes in the happer of ane grinding mill." Three times, to cure inflammatory diseases, the invocation of the three angels is repeated in Cornwall to each one of nine bramble leaves, immersed in spring water. Nine times in Sussex the snake is drawn across the "large neck" of the sufferer, after every third time being allowed to crawl about. Scotch maidens wishful to remove freckles wash their faces with buttermilk, in which for nine days silver weed (*Potentilla anserina*) has been steeped. And in cases of transmission or new birth, the number of the transmissions—either three or nine—is usually scrupulously regarded.†

Nine spar stones from a running stream, made red hot and dropped into a quart of water from the same stream, which is then bottled, is recommended to be given on nine mornings to a whooping-cough patient. "If this will not cure the whooping-cough nothing else can," says the believer.‡ Nine times should the stye be rubbed with the cat's tail; for nine nights the impaling of snails is required to cure warts. Nine days a fever patient in S. Northants will wear the lace he has obtained from a woman without giving money, giving reason for his request, or thanks for its fulfillment.§ Nine red cocks was supposed in Ireland to be the sacrifice of a witch to her familiar spirit. In County Wicklow, a correspondent tells me, the points of three smoothing-irons are pointed three times in the name of the Trinity at a painful tooth—for then, sure enough, the pain vanishes. Against blains, the Saxon leech recommends the physician to " take nine eggs and boil them hard, and take the

* Dalyell, *Darker Superstitions*, pp. 388-394.
† Dalyell, p. 117 ; Hunt, 2nd S. p. 213 ; *Choice Notes* (*Folk-Lore*), p. 36 ; see *supra, New Birth*.
‡ Hunt, 2nd S. p. 218.
§ *N. and Q.* 1st S. vol. ii. p. 36 ; *Choice Notes* (*Folk Lore*), p. 11.

yolks and throw the white away and grease the yolks in a pan, and wring out the liquor through a cloth, and take as many drops of wine as there are of the eggs, and as many drops of unhallowed oil and as many drops of honey, and from a root of fennel as many drops; then take and put it all together, and using it out through a cloth and give to the man to eat, it will soon be well with him." Of another charm the leech says "sing this charm nine times in the ear and a paternoster once."*

Nine pieces of elder cut from between two knots furnished a good amulet for the epilepsy, and nine knots on a string hung round a Lancashire child's neck would soon cure whooping-cough, but the number of knots on the blue thread by which the Orkney islander was ruined was nine.†

But though the reliance we place on nine is perhaps excessive, and the place it occupies in our history generally peculiar—for it was with nine eyes the great Lambton worm was credited, which was fed from the milk of nine cows, it was the peascod " closely filled with three times three" Gay tells produced lubberkins, and it was nine Oxford persons who saw the ghost of Lady Dudley at Cumnor,—the reverence cannot be said to have originated with us, or to be peculiar to English folk-lore. Every schoolboy knows that the hydra had nine heads, but it is more to the point to learn that an Italian author (Pizzurnus) alludes to the pain arising from stings being assuaged by the touch of nine stones, that Pliny mentions the virtues of nine knots being known to the magi, and that the people of Apulia, to cure the bite of a mad dog, would, according to Pontanus, go nine times round the town on the Sabbath with prayers and supplications. Marcellus, too, recommends the thrice three

* *Leechdoms*, vol. iii. pp. 380, 381, also cited in W. de Gray Birch's "On Two Anglo-Saxon Manuscripts in the British Museum," p. 22 (Reprinted from *Trans. of the Royal Society of Literature*, xi. part iii. new series).

† Another remedy for epilepsy is for the sufferer to creep head-foremost down three pairs of stairs three times a day for three successive days.—Dyer, *Domestic Folk-Lore*, p. 153.

times repetition of a certain verse as a remedy which experience had found to be effectual.* Three handfulls of dust saved the unburied soul from wandering by the Styx,

> Quamquam festinas, non est mora longa, licebit,
> Injecto ter pulvere curras.

In the west of Ireland in order to procure a woman's safe delivery it was customary to count over her nine articles of clothing—men's, if possible.†

Although *seven* might have been expected to be a popular number in England from its frequent mystical associations in Scripture, I can find but few examples of its use in Folk-Medicine. The Assyrians held that seven evil spirits might at once enter a man, and one tablet tells how when the god stands by the sick man's bedside—

" Those seven evil spirits he shall root out, and shall expel them from his body.

" And those seven shall never return to the sick man again."‡

---

* Pizzurnus, *Enchiridion Exorcisticum*, p. iii. c. 5, p. 55 ; Pliny, *Hist. Nat.* lib. xxviii. § 12 ; Dalyell, pp. 392, 393 ; Marcellus, *Empiricus de Medicamentis*, § 8, p. 278 ; the Apulian prayer (Pettigrew, p. 78) runs thus :—

>Alme vithe pellicane,
>Oram qui tenes Apulam,
>Littusque polyganicum
>Qui Morsus rabidos levas,
>Irasque canum mitigas.
>Tu, Sancte, Rabiem asperam
>Rictusque canis luridos,
>Tu sævam prohibe lucem.
>I procul hinc Rabies
>Procul hinc furor omnis abesto.

Five and seven are the favourite numbers in China in superstitions, but in his "Numerical Categories" Mr. Mayers gives sixty-eight current phrases with reference to the number three, and only sixty-three and eighteen with reference to numbers five and seven respectively. Dennys, *Folk-Lore of China*, p. 40.

† *Irish Popular and Medical Superstitions*, p. 13.

‡ Assyrian Talismans and Exorcisms, translated by H. F. Talbot. *Records of the Past*, vol. iii. p. 143. At p. 147 is a Babylonian charm against a magician, of whom Hea says to the sick man " by means of the number he enslaves thee."

When certain magic words are to be used against "a warty eruption," the Saxon leech says, "one must take seven little wafers, such as a man offereth with."* Although, no doubt, the wise men and women would, if questioned, say with Trickmore, "let the number of his bleedings and purgations be odd, numero Deus impare gaudet," yet the number seven was not of great healing significance save in the succession of sons, and to the personal powers of a seventh son reference is made elsewhere. A seventh son is looked upon with horror in Portugal, and is supposed to assume the likeness of an ass on Saturdays—but this is exceptional. To cure ague, West Sussex counsels say, "Eat fasting seven sage leaves for seven mornings fasting." † To cure a sore mouth, the eighth Psalm is repeated in Devonshire over the patient seven times on three mornings; but in other places, to cure thrush, it is repeated three times on three mornings. If it was said, "With the virtue," it was an unfailing cure."‡

The running, or rhyme number spells, are curious. Against the bite of an adder a piece of hazlewood, fastened in the shape of a cross, should be laid softly on the wound, and the following lines, twice repeated, "blowing out the words aloud, like one of the commandments":—

> Underneath this hazelin mote,
> There's a braggoty worm with a speckled throat,
>   Nine double is he ;
> Now from nine double to eight double,
> And from eight double to seven double,
> And from seven double to six double,

---

* Cockayne, vol. iii. p. 43.

† Dyer, *English Folk-Lore*, p. 23 : "He that would live for aye, must eat sage in May," is another saying.

‡ *Choice Notes* (*Folk-Lore*), pp. 169, 218. Some say three times every day on three days in the week for three successive weeks.—Dyer, *Domestic Folk-Lore*, p. 163. The mention of babes and sucklings probably led to its selection as a charm for children's eases.

And from six double to five double,
And from five double to four double,
And from four double to three double,
And from three double to two double,
And from two double to one double,
And from one double to no double.
No double hath he! *

Another version, to much the same effect, but actually taken from the MS. of a charmer, runs thus:—

"*A Charam for the Bite of an Ader.*

"'Bradgty, bradgty, bradgty under the ashing leaf' to be repeated three times, and strike your hand with the growing of the hare. 'Bradgty, bradgty, bradgty,' to be repeated three times, nine before eight, eight before seven, seven before six, six before five, five before four, four before three, three before two, two before one, and one before every one. Three times for the bite of an adder."†

Another Cornish charm, to cure a tetter, is:—

Tetter, tetter, thou hast nine brothers,
   God bless the flesh and preserve the bone;
   Perish, thou tetter, and be thou gone,
     In the name, &c.

Tetter, tetter, thou hast eight brothers,
   God bless the flesh and preserve the bone;
   Perish, thou tetter, and be thou gone,
     In the name, &c.

Tetter, tetter, thou hast seven brothers,
   &c.   &c.   &c. ‡

Thus the verses are continued under tetter having "no brother" is imperatively ordered to begone.

    There is a divinity in odd numbers
    Either in nativity, chance, or death.

---

* Hawker, *Footprints of Former Men in Far Cornwall*, p. 177.
† Braggaty = spotted, mottled.
‡ Hunt, 2nd S. p. 214.

A common charm for ague, to be said up the chimney by the eldest female of the family on St. Agnes Eve, is,—

> Tremble and go !
> First day shiver and burn,
> Tremble and quake !
> Second day shiver and learn,
> Tremble and die !
> Third day never return.*

A doctor's first patient, people say, is always cured, and if a person who sees an epileptic fit for the first time draws blood from the patient's little finger, the patient will be restored to his every-day health.

2. Influence of the Sun and Moon.

Mead says that "the learned Kirckringius" relates the following story :—He knew a young gentlewoman whose beauty depended upon the lunar force, insomuch that at full moon she was very handsome, but in the decrease of the moon became so wan and ill-favoured that she was ashamed to go abroad till the return of the new moon gave fullness to her face and attraction to her charms. If this were indeed the case, we can fully credit a later assertion of Mead, that the powerful action of the moon is observed not only by philosophers and students of natural history, but "even by common people, who have been fully persuaded of it time out of mind."† True it is that Cornishmen believe that a child born in the interval between an old moon and the first appearance of a new one will never live to attain puberty ; old people of extreme age are said to die at new or full moon. Galen is cited to the effect that animals born at full moon are strong and healthy. Bacon is said to have fallen invariably into a syncope during a lunar eclipse. In Sussex a new May moon is credited with curing scrofulous complaints

---
* Pettigrew, p. 70.
† Mead, *Influence of Sun and Moon upon Human Bodies.—Works*, p. 132.

when aided by certain charms. A correspondent in Rochester, U.S.A., tells me that an old black woman there asserts that asthma can be cured by walking three times round the house at midnight alone, at the fall of moon; to cure rickets, further, if you bury a lock of the child's hair at a cross-road it will be all the better if the full moon is shining.* When the moon is one day old, he who is attacked by sickness, according to the leeches, "will be perilously bestead. If sickness attacks him when the moon is two days old he will soon be up. If it attacks him when the moon is three days old he will be fast-ridden, and will die. If it attacks him when the moon is four days old he will have a hard time of it, and yet will recover. If it attacks him when the moon is five days old he may be cured. If it is six days old, and sickness comes on him, he will live. If it be seven days old he will be long in a bad way. If it be eight days old, and disease attacks him, he will die soon. If it be nine, ten, or eleven days old he will be ill long, and, notwithstanding, recover. If it be twelve days old he will soon be up. If it be fourteen nights old, or fifteen, or sixteen, or seventeen, or eighteen, or nineteen, there will be great danger on those days. If it be twenty days old he will be long abed and recover. If it be twenty-one, twenty-two, or twenty-three, he will lie long in sickness and suffer and recover. If it is twenty-four he will keep his bed. If it is twenty-five he is perilously bestead. If he is attacked when the moon is twenty-six, twenty-seven, twenty-eight, or twenty-nine days, he will recover. If he is attacked when the moon is thirty days old he will hardly recover, and yet will leave his bed."† Martius, in his Erfurt

* *F. L. Record*, vol. i. p. 45; Miss C. F. G. 28th Nov. 1879, "In Madagascar the waning of the moon is an unfavourable time for any important undertaking. Among the Antankarana the dead are only buried immediately after the new moon appears."—*F. L. Record*, vol. ii. p. 32; Cf. Grimm, *Deutsche Mythologie*, vol. ii. p. 596.
† Cockayne, vol. iii. p. 183.

address of 1700, speaking of the effect, according to rustics, of the moon's position upon the sap of growing plants, from which he says "primum nemo negabit, lunam virtute sua in corpore sibi subjecta manifesto agere," proceeds, "et observarunt medici ac chirurgi, referente Waldschmidio, non solum vulvera capitis in plenilunio ob cerebri turgescentiam majori cum periculo conjuncta esse, quam in novilunio, ubi cerebrum magis subsidet," but that all purgatives have happier issues when the moon is waning.* Mead, following Galen, says the moon governs the period of epileptic cases, and that when he had met sailors who had contracted the disease by frights in sea-engagements or storms in Queen Anne's wars, he was often able to predict the times of the fits with tolerable certainty; "and T. Bartholin," he continues, "tells a story of an epileptic girl who had spots in her face which varied both in colour and magnitude according to the time of the moon So great, says he, is the correspondence between our bodies and the heavens." Chaucer refers to a fever caused by the moon when he speaks of a blaunche or white fever in *Troilus and Cressida*—

> And some thou seydest hadde a blaunche fevere,
> And preydest God he sholde never kevere.—i. cxxxi.†

To cure warts in the west of Scotland, the sufferer is directed —instead of addressing words of endearment to the moon as would a Lancashire maid, desiring to know her true love— to stand still, and take a small portion of earth from under the right foot when he first catches sight of the new moon. The

* Martins, *De Magia Naturali, ejusque usu medico ad magice et magica curandum*, 1700, Erfurt, pp. 21 *et seq*. "That births and deaths chiefly happen about the new and full moon is an axiom even among women. The husbandmen likewise are regulated by the moon in planting and managing trees, and several other of their occupations. So great is the empire of the moon over the terraqueous globe."—Mead, *Works*, pp. 145, 146.

† For, as Mr. Fleay has pointed out, fevers were divided into red (Mars), black (Saturn), yellow (Sun), and white (Moon), according as they showed inflammation, mortification, jaundice or pallor.—*Folk-Lore Record*, vol. ii. p. 158.

earth he makes into a paste, which he puts on the wart, wrapping it round with a cloth; plaster and cloth should remain till the moon is out.*

Sir Kenelm Digby, in his *Discourse on the Power of Sympathy*, in a well-known passage asks if one would not think it a folly that one should wash his hands in a well-polished silver basin, wherein there was not a drop of water; "yet this may be done by the reflection of the moonbeams only, which will afford it a complete humidity to do it; but they who have tried it have found their hands much moister than usually; but this is an infallible way to take away warts from the hands if it be often used."†

Mead's general explanation of the moon's influence is—" If the time in which either the peccant humour is prepared for secretion, or the fermentation of the blood is come to its height, falls in with those changes in the atmosphere which diminish its pressure at the new and full moon, the crisis will then be more complete and easy; and also that this work may be forwarded or delayed a day upon the account of such an alteration in the air, the distension of the vessels upon which it depends being hereby made more easy, and a weak habit of body, in some cases, standing in need of this outward assistance."‡

It is a common superstition that it is when the tide is at the lowest that death occurs. Who does not remember the end of Sir John Falstaff,—" A' parted," says the Hostess, " even just between twelve and one, even at the turning o' the tide;" and better than many other quotations will be the familiar words of Dickens in *David Copperfield*. Barkis is dying. "'He's a going out with the tide,' said Mr. Peggotty to me, behind his hand.

* Mead, p. 132; F. L. *Record*, vol. ii. p. 158; Napier, p. 97; Invocation of Moon, cf. Aubrey, *Remains of Gentilisme*, pp. 83, 131; Dennys, *Folk-Lore of China*, p. 117; Nork. *Mythologie der Volksagen und Volksmärchen*, p. 920; Grimm, vol. ii. pp. 587-596; Livingstone, *South Africa*, p. 235; Lubbock, *Origin of Civilisation*, pp. 317-318.

† See also Aubrey, p. 188. ‡ Mead, *ibid.* p. 145.

"My eyes were dim, and so were Mr. Peggotty's; but I repeated in a whisper, 'With the tide?'

"'People can't die, along the coast,' said Mr. Peggotty, 'except when the tide's pretty nigh out. They can't be born, unless it's pretty nigh in—not properly born, till flood. He's a going out with the tide. It's ebb at half arter three, slack water half an hour. If he lives 'till it turns, he'll hold his own till past the flood, and go out with the next tide.'

* * * * * *

"I was on the point of asking him if he knew me, when he tried to stretch out his arms, and said to me, distinctly, with a pleasant smile:

"'Barkis is willing!'

"And, it being low water, he went out with the tide."

It is said, in Ireland, that if a woman's last child is born when the moon is on the increase, the next birth will be a boy, but if on the decrease it will be a girl.* The following common lines, formerly repeated by Ulster midwives after they had marked each outside corner of the house with a cross, but before they crossed the threshold, is virtually a prayer to the moon. It is still, with the alteration of the third person to the first, in use as a prayer in rural districts:—

> There are four corners to her bed,
> Four angels at her head:
> Matthew, Mark, Luke, and John;
> God bless the bed that she lies on.
> New moon, new moon, God bless me,
> God bless this house and family.†

The influence of the belief in planetary influence was seen in the constellated rings to which reference is elsewhere made; and so recently as June 1875, at the inquest held on the body of Miriam Woodham, who died under the prescriptions of a herbalist, it was elicited that the pills he gave her were made

---

* *Irish Popular and Medical Superstitions*, p. 15.
† *Lancashire Folk-Lore*, p. 69 (foot-note).

from seven herbs which were governed by the sun. A Babylonian exorcism runs, " On the sick man, by means of sacrifice, may perfect health shine like bronze ; may the Sun god give this man life ; may Merodoch, the eldest son of the deep, give him strength, prosperity, and health ; may the king of heaven preserve, may the king of earth preserve."* The Assyrians trusted in an image of Hea placed in the doorway keeping away the evil spirits. The Finns invoke the sun by the name of Beiwe, " pour le protéger des démons de la nuit et guérir certaines maladies, spécialement les infirmités de l'intelligence, de même que les Accads leur Oud, qui personnifie la même astre." A Persian remedy for bad dreams comes to me from America,— if you tell them to the sun you will cease to be troubled with them. The manifold contortions of the dervishes are supposed to repeat the movements of the planets. The devil dancers of Southern India are thought to tempt the evil spirits of the stars to enter them, and so become dissipated, instead of afflicting the people generally.†

Fracastorius could predict plague by the conjunction of many stars under the large fixed stars. Kircher, " after a strict examination of almanacs and astrological tables," pointed out the evil effects of a conjunction of Mars and Saturn, which he contended emitted both very deadly exhalations ; myriads of animalcules were generated, and such diseases as small-pox, measles, or fever became inevitable."‡ Culpepper declares the greatest antipathy to be between Mars and Venus in a passage which is as quaint now as it was once, no doubt, satisfactory : " One is hot, the other cold ; one diurnal, the other nocturnal ; one dry, the other moist ; their houses are opposite ; one mas-

---

* Conway, *Demonology and Devil Lore*, vol. i. p. 260 ; *Records of the Past*, vol. i. p. 135, "Babylonian Exorcisms," translated by Prof. Sayce.

† Lenormant, *La Magie chez les Chaldéens*, p. 224 ; Miss C. F. G. 28th Nov. 1879 ; London *Times*, June 11, 1877 ; Conway, vol. i. p. 250.

‡ Pettigrew, p. 19.

K

culine, the other feminine; one public, the other private; one is valiant, the other effeminate; one loves the light, the other hates it; one loves the field, the other the sheets; then the throat is under Venus, the quinsie lies in the throat, and is an inflammation there. Venus rules the throat (it being under Taurus, her sign). Mars eradicates all diseases in the throat by his herbs (of which wormwood is one), and sends them to Ægypt on an errand, never to return more; this by antipathy. The eyes are under the luminaries; the right eye of a man, and the left eye of a woman, the sun claims dominion over; the left eye of a man, and the right eye of a woman, are the privileges of the moon; wormwood, an herb of Mars, cures both; what belongs to the sun by sympathy, because he is exalted in his house, but what belongs to the moon by antipathy, because he hath his fall in hers."*

It was to the tail of the demon Rahu that the Indians traced, not only comets and meteors, but also diseases, and the name, Ketu, is said to be almost another word for disease.† The first time a Cornish invalid goes out he must go in a circuit, and *with* the sun; if he goes the contrary way to the sun there will be a relapse. When a New England woman will cure warts she rubs the wart seven times round with the third finger of the left hand with the course of the sun, and if she is truly gifted the wart will disappear in a few days; but not everyone, I am told, has the power to make this charm. This was the natural progression, and perhaps, as Dalyell has suggested,‡ motion with the sun's apparent course may involve a religious act in following it with the gaze from below. To move against the sun was to exhibit respect for Satan, in much the same way as repeating the Lord's Prayer backwards was supposed to do.

---

* Culpepper, *English Physician,* enlarged, pp. 266-267. See " On the Influence of the Stars," Martius, *De Magia Naturali* (cited *supra*).

† Dictionary of Böhtlingk and Rath, cited in Conway, *Demonology,* vol. i. pp. 254-255.

‡ Dalyell, *Darker Superstitions of Scotland,* p. 456.

But going "widderschynnes," as this retrograde motion was termed, was much resorted to. When Thomas Grieve, with some idea of sacrifice in his mind, took an animal to kill for the cure of a sick family, he put the animal out of the window thrice, and took it at the door thrice, "widderschynnes." This was in 1623. John Sinclair carried his sister backward to the kirk, and then laid her to the north. To cure sleepy fever in north-east Scotland, the patient's left stocking was taken and laid flat. A worsted thread was placed along both sides of it over the toe, and the stocking was so rolled up from toe to top that the two ends of thread hung loose on different sides. Three times this stocking was passed round each member of the family contrary to the course of the sun. If a member were affected the thread changed its position from outside to inside, otherwise it kept its position. When the process had been gone through three times in perfect silence the thread was burned.* When, in former times, a baptismal party were about to start on the often long journey to the church where the ceremony was to be performed, a quantity of common table-salt was carried "withershins" (the spelling varies, but the word is the same) round the baby. When the salt had been thus carried round it was believed that the child, even in its unregenerate state, was safe from harm.† Salt, of course, was in repute on account of its own celebrity; for, apart from the fact that salt, or salt and water, was applied anciently for distempered eyes, and used as a bandage for bites of mad dogs, salt was, as every reader of tales and ballads knows, a favourite way of procuring disenchantment. Noel du Fail recommends, to cure gout, that a piece of linen, which has previously been steeped in salted water, should be applied to the painful part."‡

* Dalyell, p. 457; Gregor, *Folk-Lore of North-East of Scotland*, p. 44.
† "I have conversed with an old woman, a native of Ayrshire, who had seen the custom put in practice when she was a girl."—J. (Glasgow), *Notes and Queries*, 2nd S. vol. iii. p. 59.
‡ *Les Contes et Discours d'Entrapal*, 1732, vol. i. p. 85.

The importance of time in birth, in disease, and other incidents of life, was suggested by consideration of planetary influence. If a child in China is born between nine and eleven o'clock, if his early path be rough at last he will arrive at great riches; and unlucky all his days will be the child born between three or five o'clock either of the morning or of the evening. But although such importance attached to the time of birth in the celestial empire, yet the fate of a man might be modified by his good works, for one was told " your filial piety has touched the gods, a protecting star-influence has passed into your nativity sheet, and you will come to no harm."* In Lancashire, persons born during twilight are supposed to see spirits, and know which of their acquaintance will be soonest to die; but others hold that this power belongs only to those born exactly at midnight. This perhaps arises from the superstition, common both in England and China, that midnight is a fatal period; consequently any spirit coming into being at that time might be supposed to have met those spirits which were quitting life. Not without reason, then, it would be argued they should be able to recognise what others, having no opportunity of ever seeing, could never know or recognise—the dead spirits.† It was at midnight that rickety children used to be put naked on the Logan stone, near Nancledrea. By day-time it was impossible to move the stone, but exactly at midnight it would rock like a cradle. Many a child was said to be cured.‡ It is after midnight of the seventh day of the seventh month that Canton women draw the magical water which, if used in cooking food for the patient, will cure cutaneous diseases or fevers.

* Dennys, *Folk-Lore of China*, p. 8; Giles, *Strange Stories from a Chinese Studio*, vol. ii. p. 67.

† Harland and Wilkinson, *Lancashire Folk-Lore*, p. 105; Dennys, *Folk-Lore of China*, p. 27.

‡ Hunt, *Romances and Drolls*, first series, p. 195: "If, however, the child was 'misbegotten,' or if it was the offspring of dissolute persons, the stone would not move, and consequently no cure was effected."

Such water, though kept for years, will never become putrid. Rain which falls on Holy Thursday is, in the neighbourhood of Banbury, to return to our own country, carefully bottled for use in cases of sore eyes.* So, too, in Worcestershire, a correspondent informs me, and probably generally over England, the superstition holds good. Good Friday bread, as known in the same county, is a small lump of dough put in the oven early in the morning of Good Friday, and baked until perfectly hard throughout. A small quantity of this, grated, is given to a patient when all other remedies fail. It is kept hanging from the roof.† Hot cross buns, if kept from one Good Friday to another, are thought, in Lancashire, to prevent an attack of whooping-cough. On the whole, the reputation of Friday is good throughout folk-medicine. The most favourable time to visit a seventh son is said to be, in Ireland at least, on a Friday, just before sunrise—just at the cock-crowing perhaps, which in Europe generally was looked upon as the proper time for taking medicine. For plying venom, and every venomous swelling, the leeches say churn butter on a Friday from cream which has been milked from a neat or hind all of one colour; let it be mingled with water, sing over it nine times a litany, and nine times the Paternoster, and nine times an incantation. Even for deep wounds this Friday ceremony would be good.‡

In Scotland illness was expected to be more severe on Sunday than on any other day; and a relapse was anticipated if the patient seemed easier. And yet it was a day of special healing at many wells. Sick children were carried, on the first Sunday of May, to St. Anthony's Well, near Maybole, and on that day were the waters of the cave of Uchtrie Macken, and the white loch of Merton, most efficacious, and the well at Ruthven. The

---

* Dennys, loc. cit. p. 38 ; Thiselton Dyer, *English Folk-Lore*, p. 152.

† Miss S. 8 March, 1879.

‡ "Fairy Superstitions in Donegal," *University Mag.* August, 1879, p. 218 ; Pizzurnus, *Enchiridion*, iii. lib. 1, c. 5, p. 54 ; Dalyell, p. 420 ; Cockayne, vol. ii. p. 113.

well at Trinity Gask was sought on the first Sunday of June. There appears to have been some old charm for toothache, which ran over the days for the week, for we have the following as a mock charm in *A. C. Mery Talys* :—

> "The son on the Sonday,
> The mone on the Monday,
> The Trynyté on the Tewsday." *

It was on Sunday that the people of Apulia circumvented the walls of their town nine times, to secure the cure of one bitten by a tarantula, or a mad dog.

When Shane, the son of Croohoore Bawn, was a priest in Rome, he saw one of the students shaving himself on a Monday.

> "'Mor a smoh, lath veh vuan
> Naw dane lum an Luan,'

said Shane. 'What's that you're saying?' said the student. 'Why,' said Shane, 'it's an old Irish saying; and the meaning of it is, 'if you wish to live long, don't shave on a Monday.' 'I have you now,' thought the student, though he said nothing to Shane; but as soon as he had done shaving away he goes to the abbot, and told him what Shane said, saying it was a great crime for a priest to believe in any such thing, and that he had no right to be bringing his auld Irish pishogues (charms) to Rome." † All rhymes as to the days of birth seem to agree that Monday's child should be fair of face, but I am surprised that the day of the moon should not have had more honour in the medical lore of the people. Possibly, further research may result in information on this point.

The first Wednesday in May is the day in Cornwall for bathing rickety children, and on the first three Wednesdays of May children suffering from mesenteric disease are dipped three

---

* Sinclair, *Stat. Ac. of Scotland*, 1793, vol. v. p. 82; Dalyell, p. 80; *Shakespeare Jest Books*, 1864, pp. 58, 59.

† Croker, *Legends of Killarney*, 1879 ed. p. 74.

times in Chapell Uny "widderschynnes," and widderschynnes dragged three times round the well. A ring of pure gold, inscribed with certain letters, was to be worn on a Thursday, at the decrease of the moon, by the patient of Marcellus (temp. Marcus Aurelius), who suffered from pain in the side. If the pain were in the left side the ring was to be worn on the right hand, and if in the right side the ring was to be worn on the left hand.*

Vervain is recommended for "sore of liver" in the *Herbarium Apuleii*, if taken on Midsummer Day, and lithewort (*Sambucus ebulus*) for another complaint, if taken before the rising of the sun "in the month which is named July."†

To conclude, let us note the days of danger, as the leech-books give us them. They are, in March the first, and fourth before the end; in April the tenth, and eleventh before the end; in May the third, and seventh before the end; in June the tenth, and fifteenth before the end; in July the twelfth, and tenth before the end; in August the first, and second before the end; in September the third, and tenth before the end; in October the third, and tenth before the end; in November the fifth, and third before the end; in December the seventh, and tenth before the end; in January the first, and seventh before the end; in February the fourth, and third before the end.‡ It is not so long ago that medical men stoutly defended their belief in the influence of the moon on lunacy; and that a full moon has more influence than a waning moon is still a far from rare thought of country people.

---

* Hunt, *Romances and Drolls*, second series, p. 55; Jones, *Finger Ring Lore*, p. 147.
† Cockayne, vol. i. pp. 91, 127.   ‡ Cockayne, vol. ii. p. 153.

CHAPTER IX.

PERSONAL CURES.

UNDER some such heading as this we must group those instances of cures through the merits of a special healer which are not infrequently met with. The power of a seventh son is known everywhere to be indeed remarkable,—according to a Scotch writer, if worms had been put into his hand before baptism, or, according to an Irish, if his hand has, before it has touched anything for himself, been touched with his future medium of cure. Thus, if silver is to be the charm, a sixpence or a threepenny piece is put into his hand, or meal, salt, or his father's hair, "whatever substance a seventh son rubs with must be worn by his parents as long as he lives." The former ceremony was the simpler, because the child was thenceforth believed to be able to heal by simply rubbing the afflicted part with his hand. If the child was born on Easter Eve he might be expected, according to foreign lore, to cure also tertian or quartan fevers.* There is mention in Grimm of the reputation a *fifth* son enjoys in France,† but if we may trust *Le Journal du Loiret* of some twenty-three years ago the seventh son is supreme, for he has on his body somewhere the mark of a fleur-de-lis, and like the kings of France and Eng-

---

* Gregor, *Folk-Lore of North-East of Scotland*, p. 47; "Fairy Superstitions in Donegal," *University Mag.* August, 1879 *Notes and Queries*, 5th S. vol. xii. p. 386.

† Grimm, *Deutsche Mythologie*, vol. ii. p. 964, " Nach franz abergl. 22 ist es der fünfste sohn." Cures were brought (temp. Charles II.) by Valentine Greatsakes, see letter to Boyle, or by John Leverett, neither of whom seems to have been of peculiar birth.—Pettigrew, pp. 155, 156.

land in former days can cure simply by breathing upon the part affected, as allowing the patient to touch his fleur-de-lis. Of all the *marcous* of the Orléanais, he of Ormes, says *Le Journal du Loiret*, is the best known and most celebrated. Every year, from twenty, thirty, forty leagues around, crowds of patients come to visit him; but it is particularly in Holy Week that his power is efficacious, and on the night of Good Friday, from midnight to sunrise, the cure is certain. Accordingly, at this season from four to five hundred persons press round his dwelling to take advantage of his wonderful powers.

It scarcely surprises us that a twenty-first son, born without the intervention of a daughter, should have performed prodigious cures.*

The merits of a seventh daughter are not unknown. A herbalist in Plymouth, who was tried in June 1876 for obtaining a sovereign on false pretences from a pauper, represented herself to be the seventh daughter of the seventh daughter of a seventh daughter. Nevertheless she had to refund the sovereign. In the *Superstitions Anciennes et Modernes* of 1733 it is recorded: "On me disoit, il y a quelque tems, que les septièmes filles avoient le privilège de guérir des mules aux talons." †

Those who were born with their feet first were, in the northeast of Scotland, to be credited with the power of healing all kinds of sprains, and lumbago and rheumatism. As the virtue lay in the feet, although cures might be effected by rubbing, trampling on the suffering part was most recommended; in Cornwall the merit also attached to the mother of the child who was so born, and she was accordingly invited to trample on rheumatic patients.‡ The touch of a child who has never seen his father cures swellings, Grimm says, and Bernard's *Super-*

* *Choice Notes* (*Folk-Lore*), p. 59 ; *Gent. Mag.* 1731, vol. i. p. 543.
† *Notes and Queries*, 5th S. vol. vi. pp. 144, 176 ; *Superstitions Anciennes et Modernes: Préjugés Vulgaires qui ont induit les Peuples à des Usages et à des Pratiques contraires à la Religion*, book xvi. p. 107.
‡ Gregor, p. 45 ; Hunt, *Romances and Drolls*, second series, p. 212.

stitions notes : "Mais ce rare privilège ne subsiste dans l'imagination des personnes qui veulent railler, non plus que celui de guérir les louppes, lequel on attribuë aux enfans posthumes." According to the Swedes, "Das erstgeborne mit zähnen auf die welt kommne kind kann bösen biss heilen."* In Essex, a child, known familiarly as a "left twin," *i.e.* a child who has survived its fellow twin, is thought to have the power of curing the thrush by blowing three times into the patient's mouth, if the patient is of the opposite sex. To rub warts against a man who was the father of an illegitimate child, when done without his knowledge, was thought to aid in their speedy removal. A pulmonary complaint, known in the Highlands as "Macdonald's disease," was so called because it was thought that the gift of curing it by touch, accompanied by a formula, was hereditary in certain families of this name.†

Generally in the West and Midland counties of England the virtue lying in the person of a woman who has married a husband of the same name as herself, or after the death of her first husband marries a second whose name is the same as that of her maidenhood, is extolled, and this is the more strange that one of the commonest maxims for the guidance of marriageable girls is to the effect that

> "A change of the name with no change of the letter
> Is a change for the worse and not for the better."

Be that as it may be, the little sufferer from whooping-cough is in Cheshire trustfully sent to get plain currant cake from a woman who has married a man of her own name, and in the neighbourhood of Tenbury to get bread and butter and sugar

---

* Grimm, *Deutsche Mythologie*, vol. ii. p. 964 ; *Superstitions Anciennes et Modernes*, book xvi. p. 107 (in reference to seventh daughters, *supra*). To guard against whooping-cough Donegal peasants will wear a lock of hair from a posthumous child.

† Henderson, *Folk-Lore of the Northern Counties*, p. 307 ; Gregor, p. 49 ; Smith, *Parish of Logierait, ap. Stat. Acct.* vol. v. p. 84 ; Dalyell, *Darker Superstitions*, p. 61.

from widow Smith, née Jones, who has become on her second marriage Mrs. Jones.*

It was no more necessary in every case that the special healers should be near their patients than it was for medicine men, abroad or at home, who instead of health were compassing destruction, to have their victims at hand.

A Donegal wise woman having received a careful description of a case in which (say) a splinter seemed to have got into her distant patient's eye, would fill a bowl with water and walk with it to her door. "She takes a mouthful of the water, and puts it out again. 'Na, it's no there yet,' she says. Another mouthful is taken, probably with like result; but at the third trial she exclaims 'Ay! there it is!' and shows to the messenger the small grain of iron or steel, or whatever it may have been that caused the pain, floating in the bowl of water."†

Sometimes a single word was sufficient; thus, a woman of Marton, near Blackpool, became so celebrated for her success in stopping bleeding that for twenty miles around when a case occurred her aid was called in. The men and women of Zennar were alike powerful charmers, and could cure erysipelas, ringworm, pains in limbs or teeth, and ulcerations. "Even should a pig be sticked in the very place, if a charmer was present and *thought* of his charm at the time, the pig would not bleed."‡ It is impossible to avoid thinking that the best time for witches was the early part of this century. The spread of education was not in country districts sufficiently great to discredit recourse to wise men who only insisted on such simple preliminaries as an acknowledgment of faith in the charmer's power, while it was great enough to prevent a charmer who, like Alexander Drummond in the seventeenth century, cured those "visseit with

* *Choice Notes*, p. 181; Miss G. S., 8 March, 1879.
† "Fairy Superstitions in Donegal," Letitia McLintock, *University Mag.* August, 1879, p. 220.
‡ Harland and Wilkinson, *Lancashire Folk-Lore*, p. 77; Hunt, *Romances and Drolls*, second series, p. 208.

frenacies, madness, falling evil: persones distractit in their wittis, and possessit with feirful apparitiones," sharing the fate which befel him when his fame was beginning to decline. None that I know of were like him "strangled and burnt as too familiar with Satan," though even in this year of grace there are some who, with as little real knowledge as the Chinese, who, when he was told by a Taoist priest " skilled in physiognomy," that he should be a doctor, collected a few common prescriptions and a handful of fishes' teeth and some dry honeycomb from a wasp's nest and set up in practice, have practised, and not without profit to themselves, upon the credulity of their neighbours.*

A peculiar sanctity is attached in Ireland to the blood of the Keoghs. In Dublin, the blood of a Keogh is frequently put into the teeth of a sufferer from toothache. A friend of my own in Belfast writes that his foreman, on whose word he can depend, says he knew a man named Keogh whose flesh had actually been punctured scores of times to procure his blood. " The late Sir William Willis," another correspondent informs me, " says that the blood of the Walches, Keoghs, and Cahills, is considered in the west of Ireland an infallible remedy for erysipelas."†

The cure of the King's Evil, by the royal touch, has been elsewhere fully discussed. It almost now belongs more properly to the domain of history than that of popular superstitions. I shall, therefore, do but little more in this place than mention the leading points. The question as to whether the power, which belonged both to the English and French

---

* Mention of recent charmers will be found in *Notes and Queries*, 6th S. vol. i. pp. 364-365; *Folk-Lore Record*, vol. iv. pp. 116, 117. For *Drummond's Case*, in the kirktoun of Auchterairdaur, 3 July, 1629, *Rec. Inst.* see Dalyell, p. 60.

† This passage is said to be " in a small book published a great many years ago." A query in *Notes and Queries* (6th S. vol. ii. p. 9) has, unlike most such inquiries, brought me no information as to the name of this book, or any incident in the history of the Keogh family which might have given distinction to the family blood.

sovereigns, was more ancient in the family of the former or the latter raised a discussion which, to modern eyes, seems strongly disproportionate to its importance. The English claimed for their king the sole exercise of the power Edward the Confessor had exercised, and hinted that the king on the other side of the Channel had derived it from alliance with the English. The French, on the other hand, claimed a clear inheritance from St. Louis or Clovis. Both lines sedulously exercised their powers. The ceremonial was always imposing; the court was present; the sovereign had generally prepared himself by confession, and after by fasting. In England, Henry VII. had a special Latin service drawn up for his use. The Reformation did not, to the perplexing of the Roman Catholics, interfere with Elizabeth's divine power, and even a Popish recusant, who was thus miraculously cured, was converted, and returned to the bosom of the English Church. The queen changed the inscription which appeared on the touching-piece, which Henry VII. had introduced, from " Per cruce tua salva nos xpde rede" to " A Domino factum est istud et est mirabile in oculis nostris"; and when, after her reign, the size of the coin was lessened, another alteration was made, and " Soli Deo Gloria" alone inscribed. Charles II. changed the metal, and used silver instead of gold. Sir Kenelm Digby is said to have maintained that all the security of the patient lay in this touch-piece, and that if it were lost the malady would return. Charles II. touched for the evil in Flanders, Holland, and France, when he was an exile, as Francis I. had done in Spain, as his own nephew did long afterwards in Rome, and his grand-nephew in Edinburgh. On Charles's accession he touched more persons than any previous king, nearly a hundred thousand persons, and yet " in his reign more died of scrofula than in any other." When Mr. Pepys saw the ceremony in April 1661 he was not impressed—" Met my lord with the duke; and after a little talk with him I went to the banquet-house, and there saw the king heal, the first time that ever I saw him do it; which he did with great gravity, and it seemed to me to be an ugly office and a simple one." James II. touched some seven or eight hundred sick at Oxford on a single Sunday, and a petition, Mr. Lecky says, has been preserved in the town of Portsmouth, in New Hampshire, asking the assembly of that province to grant assistance to one of the inhabitants who desired to make the journey to England to obtain the king's touch. Under Anne the proclamations of the Privy Council were read in all the parish churches, and a suffering child, who was afterwards to be Dr. Johnson, was among those presented to the queen. "That many persons so touched, and labouring under a scrofulous disposition, should receive benefit, may not unfairly be admitted, and an explanation—it is probably afforded by the beneficial effect produced on the system occasioned by the strong feeling of hope and certainty of cure. Such feelings are calculated to impart tone to the system generally, and benefit those of a scrofulous diathesis in whom the powers are always weak and feeble." This explanation, however satisfactory as regards cases of grown sufferers, cannot be applied to the cases in which infants were presented, who were scarcely likely to be affected by strong feelings of hope and certainty; and yet Dr. Heylin has distinctly stated that he saw infants touched and cured. It is possible that here it would be said it was the attendant doctor's powers which had been weak and feeble until stimulated.

Charles X. of France, who touched on his coronation a hundred and twenty-one sick persons, was the last king of whom it could be said, as of Edward—

> "How he solicits heaven,
> Himself best knows; but strangely-visited people,
> All swoln and ulcerous, pitiful to the eye,
> The mere despair of surgery, he cures,
> Hanging a golden stamp about their necks."

In 1838, failing the royal touch, a few crowns and half-crowns bearing the effigy of Charles I. were still used in the Shetland Islands as remedies for the evil.* They had been handed down from generation to generation, along, perhaps, with the story which some travelled Shetlander had told of the ceremony on St. John's day, 1633, when Charles I. went to the royal chapel in Holyrood, "and their solemnlie offred, and after the offringe heallit 100 persons of the cruelles or kingis civell, yonge and old." † At the execution of Charles many persons purchased chips of the block, and blood-discoloured sand, and hair; some, Perrinchief says, did so " to preserve the relics of so glorious a Prince whom they so dearly loved," but " others hoped that they would be as means of cure for that disease which our English kings (through the indulgence of Heaven) by their touch did usually heal; and it was reported that these relicks experienc'd fail'd not of the effect.‡ Grimm notices that the touch of queens has been deemed efficacious, and this we know in England from the historic account alone of the child of the Lichfield bookseller and Queen Anne.

In Cairo, according to the passage from Haynes's *Letters*, quoted by Pettigrew, pieces of garments that have touched the pilgrim camel which carries the grand seigneur's annual present are preserved with great veneration, and when any lie dangerously ill they lay these scraps upon their bodies as infallible remedies. Remigius is said to have seen people near Bordeaux who cured fractured limbs and dislocated joints merely by touch-

* Pettigrew, *Superstitions connected with Practice of Surgery*, pp. 153-154. I take this opportunity of here acknowledging my incessant obligations to the notes of Mr. Pettigrew on this subject, and also to Mr. Lecky's *History of England in the Eighteenth Century*. Mr. Lecky's volume needs no praise of mine, but the ample and accurate fashion in which he has treated of the Touching (vol. i. pp. 67 *et seq.*) would of itself secure the meed of approbation from students of culture which his whole work has received from the public generally.

† *New Stat. Account of Scotland*, vol. xv. p. 85; Lecky, vol. i. p. 223; Balfour, *The Order of King Charles entring Edinburghe*, MS. p. 23 (Advocates' Library); Dalyell, p. 62.

‡ *The Royal Martyr; or, The Life and Death of King Charles I.* 1727, p. 174.

ing the girdle of the patient at a distance, and in the western islands of Scotland there were women so skilled as to take a mote out of one's eyes though at some distance from the party grieved. The source of such superstition, as Dalyell has said, is probably to be found in the different passages of Scripture relative to the staff of Elisha, the handkerchiefs and aprons of Paul, persons cured of infirmities by the sanctified, and at a distance, and the like.*

We are accustomed to see occasionally in the newspapers accounts of wonderful stones which cure hydrophobia. In 1877, for example, a description appeared of a mad stone in the possession of a farmer in Kentucky. It had been found in Switzerland; an Italian took it to America and sold it to the Kentucky farmer, who in twenty-three years cured fifty-nine persons. It was said to be one inch thick by one inch and a-half long; it weighed two ounces, like bone, but harder and porous. When a person who had been bitten was brought to be treated the stone was applied to the wound, and when presumably it had dropped off full of poison it was soaked in warm milk and water and was soon ready to be used again. A query as to mad stones was inserted in *The Medical Record* of New York, in May 1880, and Prof. Charles Rice's reply, with a copy of which I was favoured (condensed), is as follows: "The fable of the mad stone may be traced back to the earlier period of the Middle Age—a time when medical men first began to leave the old beaten track of therapeutics laid down by the earlier Greek and Arabic physicians, and to study and observe nature for themselves. Yet their steps on this new ground were so feeble, and rational explanations of natural phenomena, or of newly-observed facts, were so difficult for them, that superstition for a long time afterward found a fruitful field for development. Not only were new facts discovered which were unintelligible, and were, therefore,

---

* Dalyell, *Darker Superstitions*, p. 320; Martin, *Western Islands*, p. 22; Remigius, *Dæmonolotreia*, lib. iii. c. i. § 13.

often misconstrued, but sometimes there were properties and virtues assigned to newly-discovered substances which were in direct proportion to the rarity of their occurrence or the singularity of their appearance. Among such rare substances may be counted the peculiar concretions which are sometimes found in some of the inner organs of animals, particularly those concretions which consist of mineral or inorganic matter. The first notice that I am aware of, exists in the work of Ibn Baithâr (died 1248, A.D.) 'On Simples,' who gives a detailed, but somewhat confused, account of *bádzahar*, which is our present word *bezoar*, and is, without question, the substance forming the subject of the above query. Ibn Baithâr, as he usually does, gives extracts from the works of his predecessors, and among others cites a passage from Aristotle, which, however, must be a mistake, since the contents of the passage are of such a nature that they could not have been known at the time of Aristotle. At the end of the article he quotes Ibn Djâmi', who says that 'the *animal* bezoar, or that which is found in the deer's heart, is better than the other kinds.' He fails, however, to give a description of the latter, or to mention any vegetable or other bezoars. Ibn Baithâr's description already characterises the bezoar stone as being endowed with wonderful power as an antidote to poison, and ascribes to it the faculty of 'attracting the poison of venomous animals.' The word *bezoar*, which has sometimes been written *bezoard, bazehard, bezaar*, &c., is originally derived from the Persian *bâd-i-zohr*, meaning 'the wind or the breeze of poison,' in the sense of the 'wafting away of the poison,' and therefore 'an antidote to poison.' The Persian word became *bâd-zahar* in classic Arabic, *bâdizahar* in modern Arabic, and *bâd-zehr*, or *pân-zehr*, in Turkish. I have stated above that the term *bezoar*, or rather *bâd-zohar*, in the meaning of 'a concretion found in animal organs,' did not occur, so far as I am aware of, in any published work written before Ibn Baithâr's time. Yet the word was used long before him by

Arabic and Persian authors in its original sense—'antidote to poison.' Since Ibn Baithâr himself quotes from works of authors who had preceded him, the word must have acquired its double sense a considerable time before him. After the term had once been misapplied to 'bezoar stones,' and the notion of the efficacy of the latter as antidotes to poison had once spread, the fable—as it happened with many other similar ones—took a firm hold among the ignorant classes, being handed down from one generation to another as a priceless family prescription, sometimes even accompanied by a veritable family bezoar stone. These mad stones are, in our days, principally used as a supposed infallible remedy for the bite of mad dogs, and naturally every application of such a stone to a dog bite, even if the latter would have been of itself harmless, is scored as an additional victory for the stone."* Speaking of the inhabitants of the Holy Land, Kelly says "they have a sovereign remedy, which absorbs, as they assert, every particle of venom from the wound. This is a yellowish porous stone of a sort rarely met with. A fragment of such a stone always commands a high price, but when the piece has acquired a certain reputation by the number of marvellous cures wrought by it it becomes worth its weight in gold."† The "alluring stone" of Carmarthen is a different superstition. It is said to be a soft white stone, about the size of a man's head. Grains used to be scraped from it and given to those who had been bitten by a dog, and although the scraping went on for centuries the stone never got less. The stone is said to have fallen from heaven on the farm of Dysgwylfa, about twelve miles from the town of Carmarthen.‡ In de la Pryme's *Diary*, under date "1696, April 10," is the following entry: "I was with an old experienced fellow to-day, and I was show-

---

* *The Medical Record* (New York), 8 May, 1880, p. 528.

† Kelly, *Syria and the Holy Land*, p. 127, quoted in Henderson's *Folk-Lore of the Northern Counties*, p. 165. For other healing stones, see Henderson, pp. 145, 156; Gregor, p. 39.

‡ Sykes, *British Goblins*, pp. 367-368.

ing him several great stones as we walked, full of petrified shellfish. He said he believed that they are 'greuith' stone, and that they were never fish. Then I asked him what they called them; he answered, 'milner's thumbs,' and adds that they are the excellentest things in the whole world, being burnt and beat into powder, for a horse's sore back; it cures them in two or three days."*

* *Diary of A. de la Pryme*, p. 90.

CHAPTER X.

ANIMAL CURES.

HE consideration of what appears at first to be simply animal cures is rendered somewhat difficult by the fact that those animal cures do not in most cases depend simply upon the animal association. There are other associations not easy to distinguish or to trace. Paths diverge in many directions, but I have thought it on the whole better to group cures connected with animals as far as possible together, for, apart from other considerations, a comparative light is more likely to be directed to a collection than to notes scattered piecemeal. To enter into the history in detail of the beliefs and superstitions regarding the curative powers or properties of animals which have come to us, often altered and distorted, is foreign to my purpose, and beyond the limits to which it is purposed to confine this chapter.

The dog does not bulk so largely in folk-medicine as might have been expected. A cake of the "thost" of a white hound baked with meal was recommended against the attack of dwarves (convulsions). In Scotland much more recently a dog licking a wound or a running sore was thought to effect a cure.* For a fever the right foot shank of a dead black dog hung on the arm is said to be a good remedy,—"it shaketh off the fever." The head of a mad dog pounded and mingled with wine was reputed to cure jaundice; if burned and the ashes put on a cancer the

* Cockayne, *Saxon Leechdoms*, vol. i. p. 365; Gregor, *Folk-Lore of the North-East of Scotland*, p. 127.

cancer would be healed; and if the ashes of a dog be given to a man torn by a mad dog it "casteth out all the venom and the foulness, and healeth the maddening bites." Floyer says that "mad dog's liver is given against madness." This is on the principle of taking a hair of the dog that bit you, which has been referred to above; but of the modern literal observance we have an instance in a passage in Miss Lonsdale's *Life of Sister Dora*. In the out-patients' ward one day she came upon a dog-bite upon which a mass of hairs had been plastered, and though it is not recorded whether the hairs were those of the animal which had caused the wound or of some other dog, the presumption is they were the hairs of the dog supposed to be mad. A negro superstition at Kingston used to be that certain large, black, hairless, india-rubber-looking dogs that were common on the beach would neutralize a fever if stretched on the body of a patient. Those "fever dogs," as they were called, were none the worse for the contact, the fever was not transferred but neutralized.* The tongues of dogs were said in France as in Scotland to cure ulcers, but whether by licking or medical application I have no means of knowing.† In China it is believed that the blood of a dog will reveal a person who has made himself invisible, and Mr. Giles gives a tale of a magician who was discovered by this means. It also seems to have been given as a kind of Lethe draught to what in England are called changlings. ("Now I understand," cried the girl, in tears; "I recollect my mother saying that when I was born I was able to speak; and thinking it an inauspicious manifestation they gave me dog's blood to drink, so that I should forget all about my previous state of existence.")‡ It is to this association of something "uncanny" about a dog that we owe the dislike to its howling. The dog can see more than can be seen by men. In

* Cockayne, vol. i. pp. 363, 371; Floyer, *Touchstone of Medicine*, vol. ii. p. 91; *Sister Dora*, p. 170; *Notes and Queries*, 5th S. vol. iv. p. 463.
† *Erreurs Populaires et propos vulgaires*, vol. ii. p. 178.
‡ Giles, *Strange Stories from a Chinese Studio*, vol. i. pp. 52, 184.

Rabbi Bechai's *Exposition of the Five Books of Moses* a passage tells how "our rabbins of blessed memory have said when the dogs howl then cometh the angel of death into the city;" and to the same effect in Rabbi Menachem von Rekenat's exposition on the same books we have, " Our rabbins of blessed memory have said when the angel of death enters into a city the dogs do howl; and I have seen it written by one of the disciples of Rabbi Jehudo the Just that upon a time a dog did howl, and clapt his tail between his legs, and went aside for fear of the angel of death, and somebody coming and kicking the dog to the place from which he had fled the dog presently died." In the *Odyssey* it will be remembered none knew of Athene's presence save Odysseus and the dogs. Telemachus saw her not, but with Odysseus—

"The dogs did see
And would not bark, but, whining lovingly,
Fled to the stalls' far side."

Pausonius speaks of the dogs howling before the destruction of the Messenians, and Virgil says:—

"Obscœnique canes, importunaeque volucres
Signa dabant."

" Bemerkenswerth scheint," Grimm says, " dass hunde geistersichtig sind und den nahenden gott, wenn er noch menschlichen auge verborgen bleibt, erkennen. Als Grîmnir bei Geirröðr eintrat, war ' eingi *hundr* svâ ôlmr, at â hann mundi hlaupa,' der könig liess den schwarzemantellen fangen, ' er eigi vildo *hundar* ârâða.' Auch wenn Hel umgeht, merken sie die *hunde*." Grimm says above that although "nur hausthiere waren offerbar, obgleich nicht alle, namentlich der *hund* nicht, der sich sonst oft zu dem herrn wie das pferd verhält; er ist treu und klug, daneben aber liegt etwas unedles, unreines in ihm, weshalb mit seinem namen gescholten wird." Some English peasants lay stress on the dog continuing to bark for three nights, and some German on the way in which the dog looks when he barks, for if he looks upward a recovery will be in store, and it is only if he barks while he looks downward that death may be looked for.*

To rub a stye with a tom-cat's tail has long been known in every homestead and village of England and Scotland to be worth trying, but in Northants more than this is enjoined. It must be the first night of the new moon if the operation is to be performed, the cat must be black, and only one hair plucked from its tail, and with its tip the pustule should be nine times rubbed.† To remove warts, rubbing them with the tail of a tortoiseshell tom-cat in May has been recommended. Can this in any way be connected with the somewhat inexplicable tradition that a tri-coloured cat protects against fire? ‡ A correspondent assures me that when she was recently suffering from shingles a friend offered, and in perfectly good faith, to operate at once upon the cat's tail.§ The singular remedy of cutting off one-half of a cat's ear, and letting the blood drop on the part affected, is said to have been lately practised in the parish of Lochcarron, in the North-West Highlands.‖ A New Eng-

---

* *Notes and Queries*, 5th S. vol. iii. p. 204 (citing *Rabbinical Literature, or the Traditions of the Jews*, by J. P. Stehelin, 1748); Dyer, *English Folk-Lore*, p. 102; Chapman, *Homer, Odyssey*, book xvi.; Grimm, *Deutsche Mythologie*, vol. ii. p. 555; Hunt, *Romances and Drolls*, second series, p. 166; Wuttke, *Volksaberglaube*, p. 31; Tylor, *Primitive Culture*, vol. i. p. 107. The dogs see the Mother-of-God of Kevlaar when she comes to the sick son,—

"Die mutter schaut Alles in Traume
And hat nicht Mehr geschant;
Sie erwachte aus dem Schlummer
The Hunde bellten so laut."——
Heine.

† *Notes and Queries*, 5th S. vol. ii. p. 184; *Choice Notes*, p. 12; *Notes and Queries*, 1st S. vol. ii. p. 36.
‡ Dyer, *English Folk-Lore*, p. 166; Conway, *Demonology and Devil Lore*.
§ See Chapter VII. On Colour in Folk Medicine; also Pettigrew, p. 79.
‖ Henderson, *Folk-Lore of the Northern Counties*, p. 149.

land injunction to rheumatic patients is to take the cat to bed with them—possibly with some thought that they will be so much occupied in thinking about the cat that they will have no time to think about their pains.

Hair taken from the tail of a horse—some say it should be a gray stallion—is used in Gloucestershire for reducing a wen or thick neck in females. Avicenna is said to have sanctioned tying a horse-hair round warts as a means of strangling them.* If a woman, among the old Irish, had only borne daughters and desired to beget a son, the tooth of a stallion was tied in a thong of sealskin hallowed by seven masses, and suspended round her neck. In England in the present day to cure worms a hair from the forelock of a horse is spread on bread and butter and given to the patient to eat. The hair is supposed to choke the worms.† The East Mongolians, according to Schmidt, to cure the sick place their feet in the opened breast of newly-killed horses. The inside of a horse's hoof dissolved was used by a West Kent man as a cure for ague; it is kill or cure, producing a violent sickness, from which if one recovers he is henceforth permanently cured.‡ De la Pryme mentions a repulsive draught which, when all other remedies had been found inefficacious, completely cured one Peter Lelen, who had been "taken almost of a sudden, as he was at an adjacent town, with an exceeding faintness, and by degrees a weakness in all his limbs so that he could scarce go, attended with a pain in his syde which increased day by day." No sooner had he tasted the compound—horse-dung and beer—"but that it made all the blood in his veins boil, and put all his humours into such a general fermentation that he seemed to be in a boyling kettle,

---

* *Notes and Queries*, 5th S. vol. i. p. 204 ; see Lovell, *History of Animals*, p. 79 (quoted in *Folk-Lore Record*, vol. i. p. 219).

† *Irish Popular and Medical Superstitions*, p. 10 ; Rev. G. F. S., 16 October 1878.

‡ *Schmidt über Ost Mongalen*, p. 229, cited by Grimm, *Deutsche Mythologie* vol. ii. p. 980 ; *Notes and Queries*, 5th S. vol. i. p. 287.

&c., and this it was that cured him;" it is added, "he coveted strong ale mightily." Floyer also mentions this remedy.*

Generally over England and Scotland it is believed that any directions given by a man riding a piebald horse as to the treatment of whooping-cough will be followed by satisfactory results. Jamieson says, "I recollect a friend of mine that rode a piebald horse, that he used to be pursued by people running after him bawling,

'Man wi' the piety horse,
What's gude for the kink horse.'

He always told them to give the bairn plenty of sugar candy." Among other writers the cure is mentioned by the latest writer on West of Scotland superstitions.†

The skin of a wolf was reputed a complete preventive against epilepsy both in England ‡ and on the Continent, as Grimm, "Anderwärts wird angerathen gegen die epilepsie sich mit einer wolfhaut zu gürten."§ The hoof of an ass's right foot was reputed to have a similar virtue when mounted in a ring. Jones mentions that several such rings are in the Waterton collection, ‖ and Burton of old said, "I say with Reuodocus they are not altogether to be rejected." ¶ Sinistrari mentions wolf and ass together when he refers to "la connaissance que nous avons de plusieurs herbes, pierres et substances animales qui ont la vertu de chasser les Démons, comme la rue, le millepertuis, la vervaine, la germandrée, la palma-christi, la cont-

* *Diary of A. de la Pryme*, p. 38 ; Floyer, *Touchstone of Medicine*, vol. ii. p. 97 ; see also Boyle, *Some Considerations touching the Usefulness of Experimental Philosophy*, 1664, Works, vol. i. p. 142.
† Napier, *Folk-Lore*, page 96. For a recent example see *Chambers' Journal*, fourth series, part 200 (September, 1880), p. 539. Here the person consulted was only driving the piebald horse, so that the association was still more difficult to follow than had he been riding.
‡ Chambers, *Domestic Annals of Scotland*, vol. iii. p. 53.
§ *Deutsche Mythologie*, vol. ii. p. 981 ; see also p. 980.
‖ Jones, *Finger Ring Lore*, p. 153.
¶ *Anatomy of Melancholy*, p. 456.

aurée, le diamant, le corail, le jois, le jaspe, *la peau de la tête du loup ou de l'âne*, les menstrues des femmes, et cent autres." His conclusion is curious, "pour quoi il est écrit: a celui qui sautient l'assaut du Démon, il est permis d'avoir des pierres, au des herbes, *mais sans* recourir aux enchantements."* The skin of the wolf is also reputed a charm against hydrophobia, its teeth are said to be the best for cutting children's gums, and if a person once bitten survives he is assured against future wound or pain of any kind.† According to the *Medicina de Quadrupedibus* of Sextus Placitus wolf-flesh well dressed will prevent annoyance by apparitions, a wolf's head under the pillow will secure sleep, and so on.‡ The native Irish are said to have hung round the necks of their children the beginning of St. John's Gospel, a crooked nail of a horseshoe, or a piece of a wolf's skin. The left jaw of a wolf burnt is an ingredient in a charm given in the Saxon leechbook, and even a wolf's tooth, according to Albertus Magnus (*De Virtutibus Herbarum*), gives such sovereign virtue to a bay leaf gathered in August if wrapped therein that no one can speak an angry word to the wearer. Alexander of Tralles, who flourished in the middle of the sixth century, recommends for colic, as guaranteed by his own experience, the dung of a wolf shut up in a pipe and worn during the paroxysm on the right arm, the thigh, or the hip, in such manner as it shall touch neither the earth nor a bath. §

The hare, which shares with the cat the reputation of being the familiar of witches, has naturally some virtues attributed to it. Thus, that the right forefoot worn in the pocket will infallibly ward off rheumatism is a common belief in Northamptonshire, and generally over England; the ankle-bone has been said to be good against cramp. A hare's brain in wine

---

* *De la Demonialite, traduit du Latin, par Isidore Liseux*, pp. 144, 145.
† Conway, *Demonology and Devil Lore*, vol. i. p. 143.
‡ Cockayne, *Saxon Leechdoms*, vol. i. p. 361.
§ Brand, *Popular Antiquities*, p. 339; Aubrey, *Remains of Gentilisme*, p. 115 (foot-note); Cockayne, vol. i. p. xxxii.; p. xviii.

was good for over-sleeping in the opinion of the Saxon leeches; for sore eyes, also, the lung of a hare bound fast thereto, and for "foot-swellings and seathes, a hare's lung bound as above and beneath, wonderfully the steps are healed."* "Thus much," says Cogan, "will I say as to the commendation of the hare, and of the defence of hunter's toyle, that no one beast, be it never so great, is profitable to so many and so diverse uses in Physicke as the hare and partes thereof, as Matth. [lib. iii. Dios. cap. 18] sheweth. For the liver of the hare dryed and made in powder is good for those that be liver sick, and the whole hare, skinne and all, put in an earthen pot close stopped, and baked in an oven so drie that it may be made in powder, being given in white wine, is wonderful good for the stone."† The Chinese say that a hare or rabbit sits at the foot of the cassia tree in the moon pounding the drugs out of which the elixir of immortality is compounded. In a poem of Tu Fu, a bard of the T'ang dynasty, the fame of this hare is sung—

"The frog is not drowned in the river;
The *medicine hare* lives for ever."‡

The devil's mark was said to sometimes resemble the impression of a hare's foot, sometimes that of the foot of a rat or spider. Seeing a hare was thought in Ireland to produce a hare lip in the child to be born, and as a charm the woman who unfortunately saw the hare was recommended to make a small rent immediately in some part of her dress.§

As the snake is the symbol of health, twined around the staff of Esculapius or Hygia, it is not surprising that its part in folk medicine is not unimportant. In China the skin of the white

* *Choice Notes* (*Folk-Lore*), p. 12; *East Anglican*, vol. ii.; Cogan, *Haven of Health*, p. 119; Cockayne, *Saxon Leechdoms*, vol. i. p. 343.
† Cogan, *Haven of Health*, p. 118.
‡ Giles, *Strange Stories from a Chinese Studio*, vol. ii. p. 168 (footnote).
§ Delrio, l. v., sect. 4, num. 28, cited by Sir George Mackenzie, *Witches of Renfrewshire*, p. 17; *Irish Popular and Medical Superstitions*, p. 9.

spotted snake is used in leprosy, rheumatism, and palsy, and the native doctors are said to make free use of the flesh of other serpents in their medicines.* In New England in the present day keeping a pet snake, or wearing a snake-skin round the neck, is believed to prevent rheumatism; and rattlesnake oil is prescribed by the Indians for the same discomfort, and indeed for lameness of all sorts. Serpents' skin steeped in vinegar used to be applied to painful teeth. An old man who used to sit on the steps of King's College Chapel, Cambridge, and earn his living by exhibiting the common English snake, made part of his business selling the sloughs of the snakes as remedies, when bound round the forehead and temples, for every headache. In some places they are also used for extracting thorns. Thus, if the thorn has fastened in the palm, the slough must be applied to the back of the hand, for its virtue is repellent, not attractive, and where it has been applied on the same side it is said that the thorn has been forced completely through the hand. For the cure of a swollen neck in Sussex a snake is drawn nine times across the front of the neck of the person affected, the reptile being allowed to crawl about for a short time after every third application. When the operation is finished, the snake is killed, the skin sewn in a piece of silk and worn round the patient's neck. The swelling by degrees will gradually disappear, as probably it would at any rate.†

The patella of a sheep or lamb was worn in Northants to cure cramp. During the day it was worn as near the skin as possible and at night laid beneath the patient's pillow. It was locally known as "the cramp bone." That a human patella has been used does not surprise us when we remember that the knees as well as the fingers and toes of the dead were taken from the

* Dennys, *Folk-Lore of China*, p. 103.
† Dyer, *English Folk-Lore*, pp. 157, 158; *Choice Notes* (*Folk-Lore*), p. 168 (*Notes and Queries*, 1st S. vol. iii. p. 258); *Ibid.* p. 36 (*Notes and Queries*, vol. iii. p. 405).

kirk in Lowthian by the Scotch witches when they had "danced a reel or short dance."* A decoction of sheep's dung and water was used in recent times in Scotland for whooping-cough, and in cases of jaundice. The same mixed with sulphur and porter was, according to an Irish official report of 1878, administered in that year at Youghal, Ardmore, to every child who showed symptoms of measles. This dose, locally known as "crooke," brought about another complaint which the medical men found all ordinary remedies to have no effect in stopping. In Keogh's *Zoologia Medicinalis Hibernica* a similar infusion is recommended as useful in the extreme in many diseases which are enumerated.† In Somersetshire a consumptive patient is taken through a flock of sheep as they are let out of the fold in the morning. Soon after this it is believed the complaint will gradually disappear.‡

To help weak eyes, in South Hampshire a correspondent tells me snails and bread-crusts are made into a poultice. Mrs. Delany, in January 1758, recommends that two or three snails should be boiled in the barleywater or tea of Mary who coughs at night, "taken in time they have done wonderful cures. She must know nothing of it. They give no manner of taste. It would be best nobody should know it but yourself," (this is the cautious tone to be expected, but it is what any village witch should have insisted on in a similar case;) "and I should imagine six or eight boiled in a quart of water, and strained off and put into a bottle, would be a good way of adding a spoonful or two of that to every liquid she takes. They must be fresh done every two or three days, otherwise they grow too thick." From Schröder we learn how snail water should be prepared: "Take red snails, cut and mix them with equal weight of common salt, and put them into Hippocrates his sleeve, that in a cellar they may

---

* *Choice Notes*, p. 11; Pitcairn, I. ii. 217; Spalding, *Elizabethan Demonology*, p. 115.
† *Notes and Queries*, 5th S. vol. x. p. 324.
‡ *English Folk-Lore*, p. 150.

fall into liquor; which is good to anoint gouty and pained parts, and to root out warts, being first pared with a penfield." A Berwickshire man was told to rub a white snail on a wart on his nose; he did so, killed the snail, and the wart disappeared. In Gloucestershire to cure earache a snail is pricked and the froth which exudes dropped into the ear as it falls; but Pliny recommended long ago that when the uvula was swollen it should be anointed with the juice drawn with a needle from a snail which was suspended in the smoke.* An old black woman in New England advised as a certain cure the oil from a pint of red earthworms hung in the sun. To cure a child it appears from the Holyrood Kirk Sessions Record it was stripped, rubbed with oil of worms, and held over the smoke of a fire.†

A tooth from a living fox was thought to be an excellent cure for inflammation of the leg, if the tooth was wrapped up in a fawn's skin and carried as an amulet. An Irish superstition is that a fox's tongue applied to an obstinate thorn will cause its immediate withdrawal from a suffering foot. Marcellus says, if a man have a white spot or cataract in his eye, catch a fox alive, cut his tongue out, let him go; dry his tongue and tie it in a red rag, and hang it round the man's neck; and one has only to turn to the *Medicina de Quadrupedibus* of Sextus Placitus to see the many virtues which attach to different parts of the animal.‡

To cure snake bites, it is said in Worcestershire that the warm entrails of a fowl, newly killed, should be applied to the poisoned part. The occipital bone of an ass's head is said to be a

* *Book of Days*, vol. i. p. 198; Dyer, *English Folk-Lore*, pp. 121, 157; *History of Animals as they are used in Physik and Chirurgery*, 1689, p. 34; Pliny, *Hist. Nat.* xxx. c. 4; *Folk-Lore Record*, vol. i. p. 218.

† Dalyell, p. 115 (Halyrudhons, K. S. R. 1647). See also Henderson, p. 154: "Water in which earthworms had been boiled." He mentions that a live trout laid on the stomach of a child suffering from worms is believed to be a certain cure.

‡ Cockayne, vol. ii. p. 105; Henderson, *Northern Counties*, p. 159; Cockayne, vol. i. p. 339.

good periapt, and so also a bone from the heart of a living stag when inserted in a brooch from a rivet from a wrecked ship. In Madagascar, an ancient saying as to uses of the ox apportions the different parts of the animal thus : " Its horns to the maker of spoons; its teeth to the plaiters of straw; its *ears* to make medicine for a *rash*," &c.*

Fried mice are regarded in North-East Lincolnshire as an infallible cure for whooping-cough ; the mother generally prepares the mess, for full faith, of course, in its efficacy ; and instances are recorded of the whooping-cough in due course passing away, whether in consequence of this treatment I do not like to say. In Aberdeenshire, where this cure was also known, the mouse had to be eaten with a spoon made from a horn taken from a living animal, known as "a quick hornspoon." It was also recommended in that part of the country for jaundice patients.† In Lancashire it was administered to young children for another purpose.‡ It used to be a common belief that paralysis was due to the crawling of a shrewmouse over the affected limb, and when a mouse had been caught a hole was made in the trunk of a tree and the mouse plugged up in it.§

That a child who has ridden upon a bear will never have whooping-cough is a common English belief, and much of the profits of the bear-keepers of old is said to have been made from the fees of parents whose children had been permitted to have a ride. The tooth of a bear is mentioned by Floyer, with the bones of carps and perches, the jaw of a jack, the hoofs of elk, horse, and ass, and men's bones and skulls, as possessing virtue

---

* *Folk-Lore Record*, vol. ii. p. 25.
† *Notes and Queries*, 5th S. vol. x. p. 273 ; Gregor, p. 46.
‡ *Lancashire Folk-Lore*, p. 75.
§ " In recent times in Ireland milk in which a mouse has been boiled was administered to procure barrenness."—*Irish Popular and Medical Superstitions*, p. 5.

which depends " on the earthy part which absorbs acids, and on a volatile, whereby they are fetid and anti-hysterick."* Anything that a western Indian dreams of at his first fasting may be his medicine for life, and one fortunate Indian, says an American correspondent to whom I am indebted for many curious and valuable notes, had the good fortune to dream of a great white bear. It was always his guide and adviser. One day he was in battle and severely wounded. When the enemy, however, had retired, and his brother warriors gathered round him, this Indian said the great white bear, his medicine, had appeared to him, and told him that if his friends would kill a buffalo, and give him the raw heart to eat, he should be able to rise and walk, and go with them at least part of the way. The buffalo was soon killed, and the heart given to the sick man. That day he followed the trail, supported and encouraged by the great white bear, who, though invisible to all but himself, went by his side by day and slept by his side at night. The next day the bear prescribed the tongue of a buffalo, and when this had been furnished the wounded warrior was able to keep with his companions all the way. On the third day the bear ordered its patient to eat a buffalo's dewlap, and such was the success of the remedy that he reached home in safety, and his wound healing quickly he lived for many years, till, as the Indian who told the story said, " he and the white bear went together to the spirit land."†

Among such animal cures as may surely with propriety be called miscellaneous is that recommended for earache by a

* *Lancashire Folk-Lore*, p. 155 ; Floyer, *Touchstone of Medicine*, vol. ii. p. 94: " It seems that among the Indians and Norwegians the *hoof of the elk* is regarded as a sovereign cure for some malady (epilepsy) ; the person afflicted applies it to his heart, holding it in his right hand, and rubbing his ear with it." Jones, *Finger Ring Lore*, p. 153. In Father Jerome Merolla de Sorrento's *Voyage to Congo* it is said that when the elk is knocked down it will lift up the leg which is most efficacious. It must be at once cut off with a sharp scimitar. Pettigrew, p. 61.

† Miss C. F. G. 22 March, 1880.

Demerara lady to a correspondent. To boil a cockroach in oil, and then stuff it into the ear was the remedy, but one of which my informant has not as yet proved the efficacy. An old Scotch certain cure for deafness was ants' eggs, mixed with the juice of onions when dropped into the ear.* For swollen eyes the leeches recommended a live crab to be taken, his eyes extracted, and he replaced in the water alive,—the eyes put upon the neck of the man who had need, would soon bring about a satisfactory cure. For a strumous swelling the powder of a water crab, mingled with honey, applied to the swelling would justify their claim "soon he will be well."† In the south of Hampshire a plaster of warm cowdung is applied to open wounds. The breath and smell of a cow are thought good for consumption in Fifeshire and certain parts of England.‡ A paw cut from a live mole is thought in Sussex to be good for toothache. In Aberdeenshire a man who wishes to cure certain festers will catch a live mole, and rub it slowly and gently between his hands till it dies. The touch of that man will then work a cure.§ To cure a sprain an eel-skin, wet and slimy as taken off the eel, is said to be used in Ulster.‖ Scotch boys used to wear an eel's skin round their leg when bathing, in order to secure them against cramp. The liver of an eel, according to Floyer, is commended in difficulty of labour, and is given in powder.¶ Eels are said to be sent from Lochleven to London to cure cases of deafness. The woman who was collecting the eels was asked one day if she believed that eels cured deafness. She answered, "Od, I dinna ken, Sir; but thae English doctors shud ken,"

---

* W. H. P. 26 Oct. 1878 (also *Notes and Queries*, 5th S. vol. i. p. 383); Chambers, *Domestic Annals of Scotland*, vol. iii. p. 55.
† Cockayne, *Saxon Leechdoms*, vol. ii. pp. 307, 45.
‡ Rev. G. S. S. 10 Oct. 1878; R. C. C. 25 July, 1879; W. M. B. T. July, 1879.
§ *Folk-Lore Record*, vol. i. p. 40; Gregor, p. 123.
‖ W. H. P. 26 Oct. 1878.
¶ *Touchstone of Medicine*, vol. ii. p. 91.

and no doubt they should. Warts, they say in the North, should be rubbed with eel's blood.*

The Delphic oracle recommended Demokrates to get some worms from a goat's brain, and in the *Medicina* which the Saxons adopted, a mountain goat's brain, drawn through a golden ring, is recommended to be given to a child sick of epilepsy before it tastes milk. A goat's horn, laid under the head of a sleepless man, "turneth waking into sleep," and for the bite of a snake the sufferer is told to shave off shavings of a goat's horn into three cups, and to drink, at three different times, the milk of the same goat mingled with wine.† In Scotland the blood of a wild goat, with ten drops of carduus water, was given in cases of pleurisy.‡ Cameron met a communicative friend in his journey across Africa, who told the party that the six circlets of skin on his left wrist were of elephant's hide, and denoted the number he had killed. "This induced me to inquire whether the yellow ones on his right wrist were trophies of lions he had killed, but he replied, 'Oh, no; goat's skin, worn as a fetish.' "§

Irish labourers believe that if a man with his tongue licks a lizard all over, not only will no lizard ever slip down his throat when he is lying on the grass for an hour's rest, but also that his tongue has for the future acquired the power of curing any sore or pain to which it may be applied.‖

When the Queen of Charles II. was ill, and Pepys had come to St. James to inquire on 19 October, 1663, he was told that she had slept five hours pretty well, and that she waked and gargled her mouth, and to sleep again. Her pulse, however, beat faster,

---

* Of many other things with which warts should be rubbed, see *Folk-Lore Record*, vol. i.; *pig's* blood (p. 218); *lizard's* blood (p. 219); *tortoise's* blood (*ibid.*).

† Cockayne, vol. i. p. xx. pp. 351, 353.

‡ Chambers, *Domestic Annals of Scotland*, vol. iii. p. 55.

§ *Across Africa*, vol. i. p. 100.

‖ Mrs. J. (Dublin), 29 December, 1879.

beating twenty to the king or my Lady Suffolk's eleven. She had been so ill, he adds, as to be shaved, and to have pigeons put to her feet, and extreme unction administered. So, too, in another desperate case, when in January, five years later, Kate Joyce sent word to Pepys that if he would see her husband alive he must come presently. Pepys says, "his breath rattled in his throat, and they did lay pigeons to his feet, and all despair of him." This application of pigeons to the feet seems to have been a last resource; but in France pigeons used to be applied in a variety of ways to a variety of cases. To the heads of mad people, to the side of those suffering from pleurisy, the pigeon cut open along the back was applied hot. Pigeons' blood was thought good for ophthalmic complaints; some drops of blood, let fall from under the wing of a young pigeon, would cure a wounded eye if they fell upon the wound. Pigeons' dung burned, or otherwise reduced to powder, was used in poultices with linseed, mixed with old white wine, and otherwise. Naturally what France did Scotland approved, but sometimes there seems to be excess of cruelty. At times, in the North-East, the pigeons were left fluttering in their dying agony against the dying man's feet. Early in the morning a near relative would remove the pigeons and carry them to a place "where the dead and the living did not cross, that is, to the top of a precipice, and left them." * Possibly connected with the use of pigeons is the belief that persons cannot die on a bed of pigeons' (some say game) feathers. As a Sussex man said of his friend, " Poor soul, he could not die ony way till neighbour Puttick found out how it wer, ' Muster S——,' says he, ' ye be lying on geame feathers, mon, surely,' and so he wer. So we took'n out o' bed and laid'n on the floore, and he pretty soon died then." Again, to ask for pigeons is generally thought a bad sign; it is thought to be the last craving for food. " Ah! poor fellow! " said a farmer's wife

* *Pepys's Diary*, ed. 1848, vol. ii. p. 224 ; vol. iv. p. 329 ; Bataud et Corbié, *Les Pigeons devolière et de colombier*, 1824. I have not myself seen this work ; extracts were sent to me by a correspondent.

to a correspondent of *Notes and Queries*, who wanted pigeons for a sick friend, " is he so far gone ? A pigeon is generally almost the last thing they want; I have supplied many a one for the like purpose."*

So much for pigeons. In Yorkshire, here and there, owl broth is said to be considered a certain specific for hooping cough. Swan, in his *Speculum Mundi*, recommends owls' eggs to be broken "and put into the cups of a drunkard, or one desirous to follow drinking, [they] will so work with him that he will suddenly lothe his good liquor and be displeased with drinking." In Spain, storks' eggs are esteemed for the same purpose.† The owl, however, is generally thought an uncanny bird. The Spaniard says it was present at the Crucifixion, and has never ceased to cry "crux, crux." The natives of Madagascar say it is with owls, wild cats, and bats that the spirits of the unburied, or of notorious criminals or sorcerers, are doomed to associate, and the English peasant does not think more kindly of the night bird. To carry the bones of a linnet, it seems from the trial of Elspeth Cursetter, was thought, in the seventeenth century, to secure health. Alexander of Tralles advises that a lark eaten is good, and adds that the Thracians tear out its heart while the bird lives and make a periapt, which they wear on the left thigh. When the German peasant hears the cuckoo for the first time he rolls himself three or four times on the grass, and thus secures himself for the rest of the year against pains in the back. He goes through the same ceremony, if it can be so called, when he hears the cuckoo for the first time in the year. The sinews of a vulture's leg and toes tied on with due regard to the right going to the right, and the left to the left, were commended of old for gout.‡

* *Notes and Queries*, 1st S. vol. v. p. 341; 1st S. vol. iv. p. 517 ; *Choice Notes*, pp. 43, 47.

† Dyer, *English Folk-Lore*, p. 154 ; *Notes and Queries*, 5th S. vol. i. p. 504.

‡ Dalyell, footnote, p. 150 ; Cockayne, vol. i. pp. xviii. xix.; Mannhardt, *Die Göttenwelt der Deutschen und Nordischen Völker*, cited in Kelly, *Curiosities of Indo-European Tradition*, p. 98.

CHAPTER XI.

SPECIFIC CHARMS.—(1) MAGIC WRITINGS.

TO protect her child from fairies the Scotch mother leaves an open Bible beside it, when she is obliged to go from the room where it is. So the Chinese places his classics under his pillow to scare away evil spirits. Serenus Samonicus is said to have prescribed for a quartan ague that a copy of the fourth book of the Iliad should be placed under the patient's head.* In ancient Assyria sometimes the images were brought into the sick room, and written texts from the holy books were put on the walls, and bound round the sick man's brains. Holy texts were spread out on each side of the threshold. In the course of a Babylonian curse against a sorcerer it is said " by written spells he shall not be delivered." The phylacteries of the Jews were believed to be efficacious in averting all evils, but especially useful were they in driving away demons, as appears from the Targum or the Canticles. Thus it is evident that the saying quoted by Grimm, " Christianos fidem in verbis, Judaeos in lapidibus pretiosis, et Paganos in herbis ponere," is not strictly correct, for the Jews added to a trust in stones a faith in the long, embroidered text-inscribed phylactery. A charm for diarrhœa brought to Rome in the time of Gregory the Great, and containing Latin, Greek, and Hebrew words, was to be

* Napier, *Folk-Lore*, p. 40 ; Dennys, *Folk-Lore of China*, p. 51 ; Pettigrew, p. 70.
† *Records of the Past*, vol. iii. pp. 139, 142, 148.

written on parchment, and hung round the neck of him who had need of it. Marcellus gives many such charms, which were to be written on clean sheets and hung round the neck.* Mr. Napier says: "I have known people who wore written charms, sewed into the necks of their coats if men, and into the head-bands of petticoats if women." In Africa, although quotations from the Koran worn as amulets are believed to have as much efficacy as the Bible is credited with in Scotland, or Homer in the South, they are admitted not to afford protection from fire-arms, but this, it is said, is only natural, for when Mahomet lived there were no such things, so how could the Koran protect against them now?† In Tripoli, to ward off the evil eye, a written charm used to be burnt, and the ashes drank in wine while prayers were said, and the patient perfumed with incense. A prescription written on thirteen boards, and then washed off to be given as a potion, was successful in curing a king near Koalfa, and the doctor who prepared the potion was suitably rewarded for his science.‡ Chinese physicians, if the drug be not ready that is required, write the prescription, and let the patient swallow its ashes or drink an infusion of it. This practice, Mr. Tylor thinks, may even descend from the time when the picture element in Chinese writing was still clearly distinguishable, so that the patient ate a picture, and not a mere written one.§ The European custom was to attach the written charm or prescription—here they are indeed one—to the arms, neck or body of the patient.

* *Deutsche Mythologie*, vol. ii. p. 996, citing *Meibom script.* vol. i. p. 186; Cockayne, vol. iii. p. 67 ; vol. i. p. xxix.

† Astley, *Collection of Voyages*, vol. ii. p. 35, cited in Lubbock's *Origin of Civilization*, p. 25.

‡ *Letters from Tripoli*, vol. i. pp. 168, 245 ; Clapperton, *Journal of a Second Expedition*, cited by Dalyell, p. 220.

§ Tylor, *History of Man*, pp. 128-129. Is an indication of this prescription-burning to be found in the Chinese story of the old blind priest engaged selling medicines, and prescribing for patients, who distinguishes the merits of essays by the smell each makes in burning ?—See *Strange Stories from a Chinese Studio* (XCII. " Smelling Essays "), vol. ii. pp. 139 *et seq.*

According to the curious treatise of Conrad of Wittenberg, *Doctrina de Magia*, there are two classes of words used by magicians. In the first class are Jehova, Jesus, Halleluja, Hosianna, and so on: and Abracadabra, Sator, Arebo, Tenet, Obera, Rotas, Hax, Pax, Max, Deus Adimax. In the second class, " Nomen Dei et SS. Trinatatis, quod tamen invanum assumitur, contra acerrimum summi Legislatoris interdictum, *Exod.* 20. Similiter Heptalogus Christi, Evangelium Johannis, quod vel collo appenditur, vel pani et butyro inscriptum aegrotis, potissimum vero a rabido cane vulneratis, deglutiendum praebetur, *Deum* immortalem, quanta superstitio! quantae ineptiae!"* The following charms are taken from Blumler's *Amuletorum Historia*. Against nose bleeding, " Cum trina formatione crucis, una cum trina recitatione Orationis Dominicae, et Ave Maria haec verba dicunt: Max, Hackx, Lyacx, Iesus Christus. Et his credunt profluvium sisti posse." Against the pest there is this formula:—

I . N " Qui verbum caro factum est &c. Conterat omnem potestatem inimi-
×   corum nostrorum, visibilium et invisibilium, ille ab hac domo, et habitan-
R . I tibus in ea, expellat omnem diaboli nequitiam &c. Ipsa purificet et
     santificet. Ecce crucem × Christi fugite partes adversa. Vicit Leo de
     tribu Iuda, radix David. Agios × Acheas × Agios Yschyrios × Agios
     Atheneos × Eleemosynos, Kyrie-Eleison."

Of running charms, as they may be called, we have several examples in these interesting treatises, but Abracadabra with two sister charms will be enough in this place to illustrate the nature of the superstition.

* *Doctrina de Magia*, Wittenberg, 1661, § xix ; Pazig (*De Incantationibus Magicis*, 1721, p. 22) says, "Morbi in corpore humano causas naturales, nullam vero verborum magicorum veris agnoscunt. Herbis potius aliisque rebus attribuendum est, quod benefici ex ignorantia et malitia adscribunt vocibus. Et quamvis etiam Diabolus interdum hoc fuco ludit homines, nihilominus tamen ille Naturae vim inferre nequit, sed abutitur tantum turpissime naturalibus mediis."

(1.) A B R A C A D A B R A   "Quod ad vocis huius originem attinet, com-
    A B R A C A D A B R   posita videtur iuxta quosdam, ex Chaldaicis
    A B R A C A D A B   tribus vocibus Sanctae Trinitatis . . . . .
    A B R A C A D A   Alii ab Abraxas deducunt, de quo videatur
    A B R A C A D   Seldenus. Iudaei explicant per *Fulgura Deus*
    A B R A C A   *ut dispergantur hostes* ex Psalmo Dauidico."
    A B R A C
    A B R A
    A B R
    A B
    A

(2.) S D P N Q C N   "*I. e.*, Sospitante, Deo, Perdet, Nemo, Quin, Capiet
    D P N Q C N   Nemo, et Nemo, Capiet, Quin Nemo Perdet, Deo Sospi-
    P N Q C N   tante. Similis medicina ad sedandum narium proflu-
    N Q C N   uium, praecribitur, a Marcello, his verbis repetendo
    Q C N   subter diminuendis."
    C N
    N

(3.) S I C Y C V M A
    C Y C V M A
    Y C V M A
    C V M A
    V M A
    M A
    A *

" Against a warty eruption " the leeches advised the patient to take seven wafers and write on each wafer, Maximianus, Malchus, Iohannes, Martinianus, Dionysius, Constantinus, Serafion; then a charm was to be sung to the man, and a maiden was afterwards to hang it about his neck.†

A genuine Saxon charm against wens which escaped Mr. Cockayne, and other students, has been brought under my notice by Mr. de Grey Birch, who discovered it at the end of the Royal MS. 4. A. xiv. in the British Museum. Although written in prose, it is manifestly in a loose rhythm. The handwriting was of the eleventh century.

* Martinus Frider Blumler, *Amuletorum Historiam, &c.* ciɔiɔccx. pp. 18, 19, 20.

† Cockayne, vol. iii. p. 43.

"Wen, wen,
Little wen!
here shalt thou not build
nor any holding have,
but thou shalt forth
even to the nearest town
where thou hast poor (?)
any brother.
he shall lay for thee
a leaf at thy head
(?) under the footsole,
(?) under the eagle's feather
(?) under the eagle's claw
ever may'st thou wither,
[&] shrink, as it were,
a coal on the earth;
[and] shrink, as it were,
(?) excreta voided;
and wither, as it were,
water in a vessel;
so little may'st thou become,
as a grain of linseed
And much less than
As it were a
handworm's hip-bone;
And so little may'st thou become
That thou become nothing at all."*

"For all manner of falling evils" the *Pathway to Health* directs us to take blood from the little figure of the sick man, and with it write the following lines, thenceforth to be worn as an amulet round his neck:—

'Jasper fert Mirrham, Thus Melchior, Balthazar Aurum,
Haec quicumque secum portat tria nomina regum,
Salvitur à morbo, Domini pietate, caduco,'

and it shall help the party so grieved."† When William Jackson was being measured for the chains in which, after his

* "On Two Anglo-Saxon MS. in the British Museum" (reprinted from *Trans. of Royal Society of Literature*, vol. xi.), p. 23.

† *The Pathway to Health*, by Peter Levens, London, 1664; *Notes and Queries*, 1st S. vol. ii. p. 435; *Choice Notes* (*Folk-Lore*), p. 267; see also *Blumler*, p. 19.

execution, he was to be hung, in January, 1748-9, similar lines were found in a linen purse that he carried—

> "Sancti tres Reges
> Gaspar, Melchior, Balthasar
> Orate pro nobis nunc in hora
> Mortis nostrae!"

"Le billets ont touche aux trois tetes de SS. Roys à Cologne. Ils sont pour les voyagers, contre les malheurs de chemins, maux de teste, mal-caduque, fièvres, sorcellerie, toute sorte de malefice, mort subite."*

While some taught that against the bite of an adder it was only necessary to speak one work, "Faul," and Pliny tells us of the merits of "Duo," a more wonderful story appears in Skippon's *Journey through the Low Countries.* Ferrarius, in his lectures, it seems, told of a Spanish lieutenant, who was suffering from ague, and how simply he was cured. The words FEBRA FUGE were written on paper, and one letter cut off daily; as each letter was cut off the fever abated; when the letter F was reached—for the doctor cut backwards—the ague left the lieutenant. Fifty other persons were cured in the same manner in the same year.†

Many magic writings are simply invocations of the devil. The following, written on parchment, was carried about by an old Devonshire woman, who suffered from St. Vitus' dance, as an amulet:—

> "Shake her, good Devil,
> Shake her once well;
> Then shake her no more
> Till you shake her in hell."

A woman obtained an amulet to cure sore eyes. She refrained from shedding tears, and her eyes recovered. On a

---

* Jackson was a proscribed smuggler, sentenced to death for murder at Chichester.—*Gentleman's Magazine*, vol. xix. p. 88.

† Cockayne, vol. ii. p. 115; Pliny, lib. xxviii. 5; Pettigrew (citing Skippon), p. 69.

zealous friend opening the paper these words were found—" Der teufel cratze dir die augen ans, und scheisse dir in die löcher," and naturally, when the woman saw that it was in this she had trusted, she lost faith; began to weep again, and in due time found her eyes as bad as ever.* Cotta, in his *Short Discoverie of the Dangers of Ignorant Practices of Physick*, gives the same charm in Latin, saying in this " merrie historie of an approved spell for sore eyes" that " by many honest testimonies it was a long time worne as a jewell about many necks, written in paper and enclosed in silke; never failing to do sovereigne good when all other helps were helplesse" until the unlucky " curious mind" opened and read.†

A young woman in Chelsea had a sealed paper to guard her against toothache. Her priest, evidently another " curious mind," prevailed on her to open it, and all inside was found to be—
" Good devil, cure her,
And take her for your pains."

A quack doctor, at Crewkerne, in 1876, to cure a young woman's mother, gave her a bottle of water with some thorns and a piece of paper in it, and told her to bury it in the garden. As her mother did not recover within the promised fourteen days, she took up the bottle and found on the paper—" As long as the paper and thorns remain in the bottle I hope Satan, the angel of darkness, will pour out his wrath on the person who is the cause of the illness, and will throw him on a bed of sickness, which nobody can cure, and as this water is tormented by the thorns, so may he be tormented by the illness, and as the water dries up in the bottle, so might his flesh dry up on his bones, and he shall not live over nineteen days, when he shall be taken into hell by Satan and his angels."‡

* *Lancashire Folk-Lore*, p. 87; Cockayne, vol. i. p. xxxiii. (Wier, *Opera*, p. 403).
† Cotta, *Short Discoverie*, p. 49.
‡ *Notes and Queries*, 5th S. vol. vi. p. 144.

(2) RINGS.

It is one of the pleasing legends connected with Edward the Confessor that a ring which he had given to a poor person, who had asked alms from him in the name of St. John the Evangelist, was brought back to him from the East by some persons coming from Jerusalem, and that it was found to have become all-powerful in curing cramp and falling sickness. From this arose a custom of hallowing rings on Good Friday, which were bestowed, according to Andrew Boorde, "without money or petition." An entry in the Liber Niger Domus Regis Edward IV.—"Item, to the Kynge's offerings to the crosse on Good Friday, out from the countyng-house for medycinable rings of gold and sylver, dylyvered to the jewell house, xxv s." shows that there were at least two sets of rings, silver for the common people, and gold possibly for such favourites as those to whom Anne Boleyn sent consecrated rings as great presents. King Henry VIII.'s practice was not followed by his son, but Queen Mary, at her accession to the throne, determined to revive the ancient custom, and had the office for it "written out in a fair manuscript," of which Burnet had a copy.*

As a symbol of eternity the ring naturally possessed, in the eyes of the superstitious, virtues of an extraordinary character. This would be more and more the case, if the connection of a particular ring with some eminent man, or with some holy ceremony, could be traced. Thus, a ring that had belonged to Remigius, if dipped in holy water, was said to furnish a good

* Brand, *Popular Antiquities*, p. 79; Pettigrew's *Superstitions connected with the History and Practice of Medicine and Surgery*, pp. 87, 88; Maskell, *Monumenta Ritualia Ecclesiae Anglicanae*, vol. iii. p. 335; *Proc. Soc. Ant.* 1st S. vol. ii. p. 292. The last two references are given on the authority of *Notes and Queries*, 5th S. vol. ix. p. 435; see p. 514, same volume.

drink for fevers and other diseases,* and the virtues of a gold wedding ring for curts, warts, and styes, are celebrated throughout Christendom. For sore of eyes we read in the *Herbarium Apuleii*, before sunrise, or shortly before the light go, the wort proserpinaca (knot-gras—*polygonum-aviculare*), and scratch it round about with a *golden ring*, " and say that thou wilt take it for leechdom of eyes, and after three days go again thereto before rising of sun, and take it and hang it about the man's swere (neck); it will profit well." † In Beaumont and Fletcher's *Mad Lovers* (v. 4) we have the same cure alluded to, though, perhaps, a little indefinitely. When Chilax is told, " I have a stye here, Chilax," the reply is, " I have no gold to cure it, not a penny." Rings of gold, especially if inscribed with magical words, were believed to be most efficacious in curing St. Anthony's fire. But the real merit of the wedding-ring is not because it is of gold, but because it is something which, once given, cannot be re-claimed. In the West Indies if you give a thing away and take it back, you are sure to have a stye, you will be told. In Donegal the stye would be cured by pointing at it nine times with a gooseberry thorn, which had been passed through a wedding-ring—and the saying generally there is, that any ring given in a present is an efficacious amulet, as, for example, against toothache.‡

A ring made of mistletoe is esteemed in Sweden as an amulet.§ Lilly says that the constellated rings made by Dr. Napper to cure epilepsy were highly successful. The continuance of the cure, however, depended upon possession of the healing ring being retained, for a woman who had been completely cured by the use of such a ring again suffered from fits on its being thrown down a well. When the ring was found again, convales-

* Jones, *Finger Ring Lore*, p. 141.
† Cockayne, *Saxon Leechdoms*, vol. i. p. 113 ; see also p. 351.
‡ Jones, p. 141 ; " Fairy Superstitions in Donegal," *University Mag.* August, 1879, p. 216.
§ Kelly, *Indo-European Tradition and Folk-Lore*, p. 186.

cence followed. The ring of Paracelsus seems, Boyle thinks, to have been a mixture of all metals joined under certain constellations.* Alexander of Tralles gives several gnostic devices good to wear on rings, as—a ring with Hercules strangling a lion on the Median stone, or have the setting of an iron ring octagonal, and engrave upon it " Flee, Flee, Ho, Ho, Bile, the lark was searching;" on the head of the ring an N engraved.† Monardes could make a ring which, if worn, "the pain of haemorrhoids would be taken away in the little time requisite to recite the Lord's Prayer." A head cut on green jasper, and set in a brass or iron ring, engraved with the letters B. B. P. P. N. E. NA., would preserve from many diseases, especially fever and dropsy. Rings of lead mixed with quicksilver were worn as preventives of headache.‡

Sacrament rings hold a high place in the esteem of English villagers. The manner in which the money necessary for their making is collected differs, as might be expected, but the general features are always the same. Thus in Cornwall a paralytic or rheumatic woman would collect thirty pennies at the church porch without asking for any. The parson would change the coppers into one silver coin from the offertory, then the patient hobbled into the church, and when the clerk had moved the communion table from against the wall, so as to allow a passage all round, she walked round it three times. The belief was that within three weeks after the ring, which was to be made from the coin thus sanctified, had been placed on her finger she would regain the use of her limbs.§ A woman in Northants suffering

---

* Lilly, *History of his Life and Times*, p. 53; Boyle, *Some Considerations touching the Usefulness of Experimental Philosophy* (second edition, 1664), vol. i. p. 209.

† See Cockayne, *Introduction*, vol. i. p. 18 (*Montfaucon*, plates 159, 161, 163).

‡ Boyle, *Some Considerations*, vol. i. p. 208; Jones, *Finger Ring Lore*, p. 113 (note), p. 151.

§ Hunt, *Romances and Drolls*, second series, p. 212.

from fits would collect nine pieces of silver and nine three halfpences from nine bachelors, the silver pieces to be made into a ring, and the pence to the maker of it. If the patient were a man, then the money was collected from women. Another account speaks of five sixpences collected from five different bachelors, none of whom shall know for what purpose or to what person they gave them. A bachelor is then to take the money to a smith (who must also be a bachelor), to have a ring made. That the smiths played too often upon the credulity of the people is more than probable. One, a Norfolk smith, informed a correspondent of *Notes and Queries* that the requests that he should make rings out of such miscellaneous collections were common, but that, although he supplied the patients in due course with silver rings, he had never taken the trouble to manufacture them specially and as directed. Brand says that pieces of money collected on Easter Sunday were regarded as peculiarly efficacious. There seems to be a tendency in the present day to shirk the ring, and simply to wear the shilling. Thus a Staffordshire mother, whose son was subject to fits, asked the clergyman of her parish, some six years ago, for a sacrament shilling in exchange for an ordinary shilling, which had already been exchanged for twelve pennies collected from twelve maidens, but no mention was made of a ring; the shilling itself was to hang round the patient's neck.*

Cramp rings used to be made from old coffin handles. In Devonshire it seemed sufficient to have the ring made out of three nails or screws that had been used to fasten a coffin, and that had been dug out of a churchyard. In China a single nail which has been so used is regarded as a sovereign charm; sometimes beaten out into a rod or wire, and, encased in silver, it is worn as a ring round the ancles or wrists. Grimm speaks

---

* *Notes and Queries*, 1st S. vol. viii. p. 146 ; *Choice Notes* (*Folk-Lore*), pp. 17, 36 ; Brand, p. 743 ; *Notes and Queries*, 5th S. vol. iv. p. 508. The suggestion has been made that the number " twelve " has reference to the number of the Apostles.

of rings made from nails from which men have been hanged as being worn by gouty patients on the ring finger of the right hand.*

The touch of the ring finger is generally believed to have a healing effect. The touch of all other fingers is thought to be poisonous. This merit of the ring finger arises, no doubt, from its supposed connection with heart, a tradition which Sir Thomas Browne says is not merely Christian, "but observed by heathens as Alexander ab Alexandro, Hellius, Macrobius, and Pierius have delivered, as Levinus Lemnius hath confirmed." Hence Levinus Lemnius in Lipothymies, or swoundings, "used the frication of this finger with saffron and gold," and hence he says the ancient physicians mixed their medicines therewith. But against this must be mentioned the West of Scotland superstition of the early part of this century, that only the middle finger was non-poisonous; all the other fingers were held to have a tendency to poison or canker a wound. The forefinger of the right hand is considered in Lancashire specially poisonous.†

Van Helmont had a magic metal from which, if a ring were made, it would cure many pains in twenty-four hours. To make use of the marvellous stones of which we hear, it was necessary to set them in rings. The agate has eight virtues; its third is, that no venom may scathe the man who wears it; and its fifth virtue is, that the stone taken in liquid will cure any disease. Boyle quotes Monardes as to the Indian belief that the touch of a bloodstone will stop bleeding. The virtues of jewels are not, however, much known among our own countryman, and to discuss the stories of Helmont and Boyle would be here out of place.

Sometimes the wearer of a charmed ring is also the bearer of a charmed girdle. Charmed belts are commonly worn in Lan-

* *Lancashire Folk-Lore*, p. 75; Pettigrew, *Medical Superstitions*, p. 61; Dennys, *Folk-Lore of China*, p. 48; Grimm, *Deutsche Mythologie*, vol. ii. p. 978.

† *Pseudoxia Epidemica* (1658), p 234; Napier, *Folk-Lore*, p. 99; *Lancashire Folk-Lore*, p. 75.

cashire for the cure of rheumatism. Elsewhere, a cord round the loins is worn to ward off toothache. Is it possible that there is any connection between this belt and the cord which in Burmah is hung round the neck of a possessed person while he is being thrashed to drive out the spirit which troubles him? Theoretically the thrashing is given to the spirit, and not to the man, but to prevent the spirit escaping too soon a charmed cord is hung round the possessed person's neck. When the spirit has been sufficiently humbled and has declared its name it may be allowed to escape, if the doctor does not prefer to trample on the patient's stomach till he fancies he has killed the demon.*

* Tylor, *Primitive Culture*, vol. ii. p. 124.

CHAPTER XII.

DOMESTIC FOLK-MEDICINE.

LTHOUGH it is true that all the charms I have occasion to refer to are domestic, yet there are some more particularly connected with the family circle which do not demand the assistance of any woman wise beyond her class to interpret and carry through, the assistance of which may be sought by any person. To put a piece of cold iron in the bed of a labouring woman to guard against fairies did not require the services of any one outside the cottage; and to ring the church bells to expedite childbirth was no hard labour for the expectant mother's friends. The tribes of the Malay Peninsula light fires to keep away the evil spirits, and the numerous notices in the folk-lore of all countries of magic stones, holy girdles, and other nurses' specials, attest the common sympathy of the human race.*

The custom of the "couvade," where the husband at childbirth undergoes medical treatment, is curiously perpetuated in Ireland. Historically the custom is traced to the time when succession through the father, instead of through the mother, as originally, was adopted. The father then became the important

---

* Livinius, in Erasmus' *Colloquies*, p. 27, says: "Do not slight my present; it is the eagle stone; it is good for woman with child; it is good to bring on their labour." See also Tylor, *Primitive Culture*, vol. ii. p. 147; *Diary of A. de la Pryme*, p. 90; Noel du Fail, *Les Contes et Discours d'Entrapel*, vol. i. p. 82.

relation.* In course of the progress of civilization, however, the father became weary of the senseless confinement and limited regimen which his position as begetter of his child was supposed to entail. The Tamil jokes the Korovan on his eating assafœtida when his wife lies-in in the present day, and most peoples have forgotten the singular practice which marked the great social and legal change. But in Ireland a tradition remains. The husband does not indeed pretend to suffer the pains of labour, but the nurses boast that they possess the power of transferring the sufferings to him or to any other person they please. Literally, in earlier times when the nurse announced to the husband that he was about to be a father she brought the pretended pains, for her appearance was tantamount to a declaration that his confinement and restricted living must commence. Now the nurse threatens a real transfer, and, not understanding why the husband should be the only sufferer, she boasts of being able to give the mother's pain to any man, particularly, my informant says, to old bachelors.†

An Ulster superstition is that each child a woman bears costs her a tooth;‡ it is probably thought a small price. When the child is born the care taken of its first days in every nation is very great. To wash a child before its forehead has been touched by holy water is thought in the Tyrol to be highly injurious to it. In Scotland the newly-born child in the Highlands was given ash-sap at once, because it is a powerful astringent and also a guard against witches; and in the Lowlands bathed in salted water, made to taste it three times, because the water was strengthening

---

* Lubbock, *Origin of Civilization*, pp. 15, 154 : "As soon as the change was made, the father would take the place previously held by the mother, and he, instead of she, would be regarded as the parent. Hence, on the birth of a child, the father would naturally be very careful what he did, and what he ate, for fear the child should be injured." See also Tylor, *Primitive Culture*, vol. i. p. 76.
† *Irish Popular and Medical Superstitions*, p. 13.
‡ W. H. P. 26 October, 1878.

and also obnoxious to a person with the evil eye.* "Amazing toughness of popular tradition!" says Mr. Kelly, writing of the Highland practice. " Some thousands of years ago the ancestors of this Highland nurse had known the *Fraxinus ornus* in Arya, or on their long journey thence through Persia, Asia Minor, and the South of Europe, and they had given its honey-like juice as divine food to their children; and now their descendant, imitating their practice in the cold North, but totally ignorant of its true meaning, puts the nauseous sap of her native ash into the mouth of her hapless charge, because her mother, and her grandmother, and her grandmother's grandmother, had done the same thing before her."†

In the parish of Culdaff, county Donegal, an infant at its birth is forced to swallow spirits, and is immediately afterwards suspended by the upper jaw on the nurse's forefinger.‡ It is a general belief that it is unlucky to take a baby downstairs before it goes up, and many have been the devices to save the infant from the unluck which might follow it. A nurse in the West Riding placed a chair on the dressing-table, and climbed with the baby to the top, exclaiming, "There, bless its little heart, it shall not go downstairs first." A nurse in the West of Scotland found a substitute in going up three steps of a ladder, but, near Glasgow, the mother was sometimes compelled to go up also. §

The German peasant will not lend anything out of his house until his new-born child is baptized. Here, of course, the fear is that evil may be brought on the child through some magic tampering with a lent article. Every one knows how unlucky

---

* Grohman, *Tyrol and the Tyrolese*, p. 56; *Choice Notes (Folk-Lore)*, p. 24; Napier, *Folk-Lore*, p. 30.

† Kelly, *Indo-European Folk-Lore*, p. 145.

‡ W. H. P.: "Many children die when one or two days old of the trismus nascentium, or jaw fall, a spasmodic disease peculiar to tropical climates; here, however, it is probably a dislocation caused by the above-mentioned barbarous practice."

§ *Notes and Queries*, 5th S. vol. x. pp. 205, 255; Napier, *Folk-Lore*, p. 31: " The late Mortimer Collins going at the age of thirteen to see a newly-born cousin

it is to cut a child's nails before it is a year old (then will he be a thief), how undesirable it is that the upper teeth should be cut before the lower, and that until the child is three months old it should be allowed to look into a looking-glass. A common superstition is, that a newly-born child should not be weighed, but in New England they say you may weigh it if you like, but by no means measure it. To measure it is to measure it for its coffin.

In Scotland it was thought unlucky to name a child before its baptism; if any one inquired the baby's name the answer was, " It has not been out yet." As the doctrine of the damnation of the unbaptized was thoroughly accepted, every effort was made to have the christening as soon as possible, and Mr. Napier says he has known of an instance in which the baby was born on a Saturday and carried two miles to church next day. It was dangerous to risk a week's delay. To decline the present of bread and cheese and salt from the christening party was tantamount to wishing evil to the child. It is lucky for the child to cry at baptism, otherwise he is too good to live. It is thought unlucky in Worcestershire to have a boy and girl christened at the same time, they will not have issue; and if the girl is christened before the boy she will be masculine and he feminine in character as they grow up.[*] It is said in Ulster that it makes a " crowe " of a child, *i. e.*, dwarfs it, if a man puts his leg over the child's head. As an antidote to sickness the Chinese stain the foreheads of their children with cinnebar or vermilion on the fifth day of the fifth month, and a medicated cake prepared at noon of the day is in high repute for the cure of diseases.[†]

(Mr. Henry Frowde, the London manager of the Oxford University Press), insisted on carrying him upstairs in accordance with the old legend." *Notes and Queries*, 5th S. vol. x. p. 276.

[*] *Folk-Lore*, pp. 30 *et seq.*; *Notes and Queries*, 5th S. vol. iii. p. 424; *Choice Notes* (*Folk-Lore*), p. 25.

[†] W. H. P. 26 Oct. 1878; Dennys, *Folk-Lore of China*, p. 70.

A Durham precaution against whooping-cough was followed by fatal results in the end of the year 1879. In order to secure her newly-born child against whooping-cough the mother's "friends" compelled her on the day after the birth to sit up in bed with the child in her arms whilst they combed her hair, so as to fall over the infant. The woman was thought to be progressing satisfactorily till then, but the next day she died.*

A curious Irish remedy for sore throat is to apply salt herring to the feet. The touch of a woman's dress is thought in China to be efficacious in cases of swelling. The garment should be applied three times. If you just place your shoes with the toes just peeping from beneath the coverlet, Lancashire people will tell you you need not fear cramp. Many people I know carry brimstone about their person as a remedy for cramp. To carry a raw potato or a loadstone in the pocket is a general charm against rheumatism. Leaning against a pair of bellows is said in West Sussex to be a fine thing for rheumatism. A coal-rake will keep away nightmare ; at least, two years ago, when a husband and wife were charged at Bradford with quarrelling, the woman stated the reason why she kept a coal-rake in her bedroom was that she suffered from nightmare, and had been informed it would keep the nightmare away. Water in which flint arrowheads have been bathed are said in Cornwall to cure diseases. Pebbles of hard chalk found on the Ulster coast are worn to ward off illness, and to go between the sun and the sky to a place where the dead and the living cross (a ford), and lift a stone from it with the teeth, is thought in the North-East of Scotland a cure for toothache. The adder stone used to be worn by children of people of good education for whooping-cough. To rub the patient's head, in case of ringworm, with a silver watch, was sometimes recommended, or the diseased part might be measured and then rubbed with a shilling. To put on in jest

* *Durham County Advertiser*, 12 December, 1879.

mourning garments will cause the thoughtless wearer, if a New England superstition be right, to die within the year of the same disease of which the person died for whom the mourning is worn. In South Hampshire the snuff of a tallow-candle is given upon sugared bread and butter to ague patients to eat. Change of air is ordered by all doctors, but occasionally their patients do not understand them. They understand that any change of air will be beneficial, if the trouble is whooping-cough, for example; they say it will "break the cough." Thus, I have known, in Glasgow, of children being taken to gasworks and to distilleries, and I have heard of an Ulster mother putting a can of coal tar under the patient's bed to cause "a change of air." A curious custom in co. Clare, vouched for by a correspondent of the *East Anglican*, was to send the town band frequently to play in the evening in the cottage of a young woman afflicted with St. Vitus' dance, with the view of curing her. Some recollection of the tarantula is here.

In Staffordshire, hanging an empty bottle up the chimney is thought a useful thing in cases of illness. To cure colic, in Towednack, in Cornwall, they advise you to stand on your head for a quarter of an hour. For poison this was a common remedy in olden times, the belief being that the poison would run out by the eyes—" Man hieng den kranken an den beinen auf, and riss ihm nach einer weile ein aug aus, im glauben, das gift werde durch diese öfnung fliessen: 'tamen intoxicatus Albertus in Austria, et diu per pedes suspensus, oculum perdens evasit.'" The Saxons said, if a man had eaten wolf's-bane, and had been duly placed on his head, some one should strike him many scarifications on the shanks, then the venom departs out through the incisions.* The common remedy for nose-bleeding, viz., slipping a key down between the clothes and the skin, has been said to be a relic of a symbolic act of the Norse, and connected

---

* Grimm, vol. ii. p. 984 ; Cockayne, vol. ii. p. 155.

with Thor, but whether assisted by faith in legend or not, the application of the cold metal is generally successful, as it causes a stoppage of the bleeding by acting in a reflex manner on the nerves, and producing contraction of vessels distributed in the neighbourhood of these nerves.

Fasting spittle is generally supposed to be poisonous, and yet it is credited with great virtues. To spit three times in the face of a man with an evil eye will counteract its influence; rubbing warts night and morning with fasting spittle will remove them. The new shilling which is to cure ringworm should be spat on fasting. Galen says that a person killed a scorpion simply by spitting. "Two old-fashioned ladies we know (they are Scotch by the way)," writes a correspondent, "hold firmly to the belief that it is very hurtful to swallow the saliva that is in the mouth on first waking. They would not do it on any account." In Madagascar this first spittle in the morning is called ròra mafàitra, "bitter or disagreeable saliva," and has medicinal virtue in healing a sore ear or eye. Marcellus says that to cure gout the patient before getting out of bed in the morning should spit on his hand, and rub all his sinews therewith, saying, "flee, gout, flee." *

For pains in the joints the leechbook prescribes this incantation, "Malignus obligavit; angelus curavit, dominus salvavit," and to spit on the joint. "It will soon be well with him." But as Dalyell says the most noted application of the human saliva by the ancients was for the restoration of sight. Hilarion cured a woman in Egypt by spitting in her eyes. Vespanian so cured a blind man of Alexandria. Captain Cook attempted to do so in the north-west coast of America. The fasting spittle of a woman after her first child, or of a woman who has borne only sons,

* *Lancashire Folk-Lore*, p. 69; *English Folk-Lore*, p. 166; Gregor, *Folk-Lore of Northern Counties*, p. 47; Dalyell, *Darker Superstitions of Scotland*, p. 46 (Galen, *de Simplicium Medicamentorum Facultatibus*, lib. x. c. 16); Miss M. L. B. 23 Oct. 1878; *Folk-Lore Record*, vol. ii. p. 36.

cured, Pliny says, bloodshot eyes.* Philagrios, in the fourth century, disapproved of uttering barbarous names when one spat into the drug pot, for without the names the spittle would be quite as efficacious in the medicine. Spittle was an ingredient in a holy salve of the Saxons.†

To cure warts a common remedy is to tie as many knots on a hair as there are warts and throw the hair away. Six knots of elderwood are used in a Yorkshire incantation to ascertain if beasts are dying from witchcraft. Marcellus commended for sore eyes that a man should tie as many knots in unwrought flax as there are letters in his name, pronouncing each letter as he worked, this he was to tie round his neck.‡ Grimm says, "gichtsegen werden in ungebleichter leinwand mit leinenen fäden *ohne* knoten auf der brust getragen."§ When Marduk wishes to comfort a dying man, his father Hea says, " Go—

> " Take a woman's linen kerchief
> bind it round thy left hand ! loose it from the left hand !
> Knot it with seven knots : do so twice :
> Sprinkle it with bright wine :
> bind it round the head of the sick man :
> bind it round his hands and feet, like manacles and fetters.
> Sit round on his bed :
> sprinkle holy water over him.
> He shall hear the voice of Hea.
> Davkina shall protect him !
> And Marduk, Eldest Son of heaven, shall find him a happy habitation."‖

The Jewish phylactery was tied in a knot, but more generally knots are found in use to bring about some enchantment or disenchantment. Thus in an ancient Babylonian charm we have—

---

* Cockayne, vol. ii. p. 323 ; Dalyell, p. 77. "So many cures are confidently averred and recorded, that it would be a most interesting topic of investigation whether any solvent sanative or medicament lost to modern oculists was not known of old."—p. 74.
† Cockayne, vol. i. p. xvi. ; vol. iii. p. 25.
‡ Henderson, pp. 139, 219 ; Cockayne, vol. i. p. xxix.
§ Grimm, *Deutsche Mythologie*, vol. ii. p. 978.
‖ *Records of the Past*, vol. iii. p. 141.

"Merodoch, the son of Hea, the prince, with his holy hands cuts the knots."

That is to say he takes off the evil influence of the knots.*

So, too, witches sought in Scotland to compass evil by tying knots. Witches, it was thought, could supply themselves with the milk of any neighbours' cows if they had a small quantity of hair from the tail of each of the animals. The hair they would twist into a rope, and then a knot would be tied on the rope for every cow who had contributed hair. Under the clothes of a witch who was burnt at St. Andrews, in 1572, was discovered " a white claith, like a collore craig, with stringis, whereon was mony knottis vpon the stringis of the said collore craig." When this was taken from her, with a prescience, then wrongly interterpreted, she said, " Now I have no hope of myself." " Belyke scho thought," runs the contemporary account, "scho suld not have died, that being vpon her," but probably she meant that to be discovered with such an article in her possession was equivalent to the sentence of death. So lately as the beginning of the last century two persons were sentenced to capital punishment for stealing a charm of knots, made by a woman as a device against the welfare of Spalding of Ashintilly. Owing to a supposed connection which the witches knew between the relations of husband and wife and the mysterious knots, the bridegroom, formerly in Scotland and to the present day in Ireland, presents himself occasionally, and in rural districts, before the clergyman, with all knots and fastenings on his dress loosened, and the bride, immediately after the ceremony is performed, retires to be undressed, and so rid of her knots.

"What admission we owe unto many conceptions concerning right and left," says Sir Thomas Browne, "requireth circumspection. That is, how far we ought to rely upon the remedy in Kiranides, that is, the *left* eye of an hedge-

---

* Chambers, *Popular Rhymes*, p. 111 ; Kelly, *Curiosities*, p. 230 ; Dalyell, pp. 302, 307 ; *Irish Popular and Medical Superstitions*, p. 4.

hog fried in oil to procure sleep, and the *right* foot of a frog in deer's skin for the gout, or that, to dream of the loss of *right* or *left* tooth presageth the death of male or female kindred, according to the doctrine of Artemidorus. . . . . And, lastly, what substance there is in that auspicial principle and fundamental doctrine of arialation that the *left* hand is ominous, and that good things do pass sinistrously upon us, because the *left* hand of man respected the right hand of the gods which handed their favours unto us."* Let us first see what can be said in folk-lore for the right hand, and then consider the evidence in favour of the left.

When black hellebore was to be gathered, the person clad in white, and bare-footed, who had to offer the sacrifice of bread and wine, plucked the hellebore with the right hand, and then, covering it with his robe secretly, conveyed it to the left hand. Pulling a plant while resting on the right knee was held in the Orkneys, in the beginning of the seventeenth century, as partaking in divination. To have warts on the right hand betokened, in the West of Scotland, future riches; and in Nottinghamshire a mole on the upper side of the right temple of a woman, above the eye, signified good and happy fortune by marriage. It is a Dorsetshire belief that the bishop's right hand is lucky at a confirmation and the left unlucky.†

To secure yourself from toothache, you will be told in Sussex to be careful always to put on the right stocking before the left, and to put the right leg into the trousers before the left. But in Shropshire, and elsewhere, exactly the contrary is enjoined.‡ After all does it come to this ignominous ending, that the one preservative is exactly as valuable as the other? In the

---

* *Vulgar Errors*, 1658, p. 244.
† Pliny, *Nat. His.* lib. xxiv. c. 11; Pettigrew, *Superstitions*, p. 23; Dalyell, p. 127; Napier, p. 97; *English Folk-Lore*, p. 280; *Notes and Queries*, 1st S. vol. vi. p. 601; *Choice Notes (Folk-Lore)*, p. 25.
‡ *Notes and Queries*, 5th S. vol. iii. p. 465.

early part of this century the Mexicans took medicine with the right hand if they were to benefit the liver, and with the left hand if for the kidneys. To hold the chin in the right hand during divine service was of old thought superstitious, and the canon law declared against the remedy of holding the left thumb in the right hand as also superstitious.* In Madagascar the right foot must always be used on first entering a house, especially a royal house. To hear the cuckoo for the first time for the year on the right hand is accounted lucky in Cornwall, and to pull off the right stocking, when the cuckoo is heard, and search on the sole of the right foot for the hair which should be there, is enjoined in Ireland and in Rome. The ancient Irish, if Gerald Cambrensis is to be trusted, did not dip the right arms of their children into the water at baptism; they thought thus to secure extra strength to the unhallowed hand. For the cure of toothache Martius recommended that the bone of the right thigh should be used to rub the aching part. The pain would cease.† Burton says of the stone called "chelidonius," found in the stomach of a swallow, "if it is lapped in a fair cloth, and tied to the right arm, will cure lunatics, madmen, make them amiable and merry." ‡

It is, however, from the *left* arm that an Aberdeenshire man would direct blood to be let on the first attack of epilepsy. It was on his left arm that the sorcerer of Sistrans always carried the consecrated host which he had stolen. Pliny tells of a wasp or beetle, caught with the left hand, being used medicinally; to plait a cord with the left hand would keep out Scotch witches.§

---

* Hardy, *Travels in Mexico*, 1825-8, p. 417 ; Dalyell, pp. 128, 447. At the latter reference citations from Martin de Arles, St. Augustine, and Gratian (*Decretalia, causa* xxvi. *quaest.* 2), will be found.

† *Folk-Lore Record*, vol. ii. pp. 37, &c ; *Choice Notes*, p. 90 ; Brand, *Popular Antiquities*, p. 339 ; Martius, p. 32.

‡ *Anatomy of Melancholy*, p. 435.

§ Gregor, p. 45 ; *Tales and Legends of Tyrol*, p. 69. Tying a garter round the left leg below the knee is said to keep off cramp.

In the *Medicina de Quadrupedibus* of Sextus Placitus, as in the Anglo-Saxon (but not in the Latin MS. Harl. 4986, nor edition, 1538), is the following:—" For flux of blood when to all men the moon is seventeen nights old, after the setting of the sun, ere the uprising of the moon, come to the tree which is hight morbeam, or *mulberry tree*, and from it take an apple, *that is a berry*, with thy left hand with two fingers, that is, with the thumb and the ring finger a white apple, *or berry*, which as yet is not ruddy," and so on. In a fit of convulsion, or shortness of breath, to hold the left thumb with the right hand was thought advice not to be despised, and a New England recipe speaks of rubbing a wart seven times with the third finger of the left hand at a new moon. When gout was to be cured Alexander of Tralles directed that it was with the thumb and third finger of the left hand that the henbane was to be dug up, when the moon was in Aquarius or Pisces, before the charm was said. This was the charm:—" I declare, I declare holy wort, to thee; I invite you to-morrow to the house of Fileas, to stop the rheum of the feet of M. or N., and say, I invoke Thee, the great name Jehovah, Sabaoth, the God who steadied the earth, and stayed the sea, the filler of flowing rivers, who dried up Lot's wife, and made her a pillar of salt, take the breath of thy mother earth and her power, and dry the rheum of the feet or hands of N. or M."*

In Madagascar, when mourning for a deceased relation is laid aside, the youngest son or daughter, by the custom known as *mitendrilo*, puts a little grease on the left side of the neck by the little finger of the left hand. To cure a burnt finger Worcestershire people tell you you should keep it secret, spit on the finger, and press it behind the left ear. For erysipelas on man or horse, the leeches would have a charm sung thrice nine times, at evening and morning, over the man's head, and into the horse's left ear as it should in running water, with its head

* Cockayne, vol. i. p. 331; Brand, p. 502; Cockayne, vol. i. pp. xix. xx.

against the stream. When a horse was elf-shot, among other things his owner should prick a hole in its left ear in silence.*

If when one hears a dog howl he is disturbed (as if he is at all superstitious he should be), then should he take his left shoe off, spit upon the sole, place the shoe on the grate with the sole upwards and place his hand on the place he sat on when the dog howled. This simple ceremony, it is gratifying to know, will not only save him from harm but stop the howling of the dog. Marcellus in the fourth century of the Christian era said to escape pain in the stomach one should always put on his left shoe first and wear on gold leaf,

L * M Θ R I A

three times written.† When the Highland shepherds kept the dogs from passing between the pair that were to be married they also looked narrowly to see that the bridegroom's left shoe was without buckle or latchet, that all the secret influences of witches might be frustrated. So, too, whether the marriage was at court or in a country kitchen, it was the bride's left shoe which was flung, with "many other pretty sorceries."‡ The sole of the left shoe of a person of the same age but of opposite sex to the patient if reduced to ashes and administered to the patient will cure St. Anthony's fire.§ Nephrite, Boyle says, should be bound on the pulse of the left hand.‖

Sometimes there is a discrimination between the parts affected and right and left. Thus in Worcestershire to cure nose-

* *Folk-Lore Record*, vol. ii. p. 39 ; Miss E. S. 8 March, 1879 ; Cockayne, vol. iii. p. 71 ; vol. ii. p. 291.

† *English Folk-Lore*, p. 101 ; Cockayne, vol. i. p. xxxi.

‡ " The Bride was now laid in her Bed,
 Her *left* leg Ho was flung ;
 And Geordy Gil was fidgen glad
 Because it hit Jean Gun."
 Allan Ramsay, 1721; Brand, pp. 398, 399, 401.

§ " I have seen it applied with success, but I suppose its efficacy is due to some astringent principle in the ashes."—*Choice Notes* (*Folk-Lore*), p. 37.

‖ Boyle, *Some Considerations*, &c. p. 206.

bleeding from the right nostril the healer will make a bow to the sufferer and press the little finger of his right hand, and if it is the left nostril that bleeds he will bow and press the little finger of the left hand. For pain and pricking in the eye the Saxons bound the right eye of a hound over the right eye of the man if it was that eye which troubled him, or the left eye over the man's left eye if necessary; and if a man chanced to swallow an insect of male kind the proper charm was to be sung into his right eye, whereas if he had swallowed an insect of female kind it should be sung in his left ear.*

Had I any intention to go at length into *plant* charms it would not of course have been in so backward a place that I should have put anything relating to a subject so important; and even as regards the few, but perhaps representative, notes which follow I may remind the reader that in dealing with such charms as are connected with plants there is peculiar need of caution. To suppose that because the use of a certain herb is recommended by a woman credited with superstitious practices, the use of the herb must be superstitious, would be to draw a conclusion little warranted by the facts. At the same time to accept all herbal prescriptions as containing the sum of knowledge of more than one generation of healers would not only be likely to lead to conclusions as erroneous, but to ignore the fact that in many cases the herb was only the accompaniment of magical words. There may have been merit in the plant in this case, or there may not have been. It was not necessary that it should have healing virtues; its merit lay in its emphasising the charm. This is not the place to consider how far the leeches old and new are right in recommending the plants they name, nor would I feel justified in undertaking such considerations at any time. It will be sufficient if I indicate the nature of the majority of the plant remedies on which reliance has been placed, and

* Miss E. S. 8 March, 1879; Cockayne, vol. i. p. 371; vol. iii. p. 11.

the customs which were associated with them. Completeness I cannot and do not claim.

"O, who can tell
The hidden powre of herbes and might of magic spell?"

says Spenser.

"Elder," says Sir Thomas Browne, "is become a famous medicine in quinsies, sore throats, and strangulations." Culpepper speaks of it curing the bites of adders and mad dogs. Blochwick mentions a cross of elder and the sallow "mutually inwrapping one another" being hung round children's necks, and an amulet against erysipelas made of elder on which the sun never shined. "If the piece betwixt the two knots be hung about the patient's neck it is much commended. Some cut it in little pieces and sew it in a knot in a piece of a man's shirt, which seems superstitious." The green piece of the inner bark of the elder was used in the northern counties for anointing the eyes, and was obnoxious to witches.* In Denmark the elder is good against toothache or fever: "Der fieberkranke steckt, ohne ein wort dabei zu sprechen, einen fliederzweig in die erde. Da bleibt das fieber am flieder haften, and hängt sich dann an den, der züfällig über die stätte kommt." Again, "besonders ist flieder heilsam des über bienenstöcken wächst; man schält seinen bast nach oben (nicht nach unten) zu, and gibt den kranken den absud zu trinken."†

A labourer's wife who suffered from ague was recommended by a charmer to bid her husband tie a handful of common groundsel in her bosom while he (the charmer) said certain incantations. Watercress laid against warts was said by the Saxon leeches to work a cure. An Irish cure for sore throat is to tie cabbage-leaves round the throat, and the juice of cabbages

---

* *Vulgar Errors*, vol. i. p. 215 (1852); *English Physician Enlarged*, 1684, p. 2; Blochwick, *Anatomic of the Elder*, 1665, p. 54; Pettigrew, *Superstitions connected with Medicine and Surgery*, pp. 61, 79; Henderson, pp. 219 *et seq.*

† Grimm, *Deutsche Mythologie*, vol. ii. p. 979.

taken with honey was said in England to cure hoarseness or loss of voice.* A chestnut begged or stolen is a preservative against rheumatism. So is a potato, and I know a gentleman who carries one always with him. He told me that he did not know whether it was superstition or not, but whenever by accident he left his potato at home he was sure to feel a twinge of rheumatism. Some recommend a double hazel nut to be carried in the pocket against toothache. Scalds are cured in Derbyshire by putting raw potato on the scalded part; and hot boiled potato is applied to corns.

A certain cure against deafness was said to be ants' eggs mixed with the juice of onions dropped into the ear. This was a Scotch recipe. In England we have the juice of onions recommended, but no mention made of ants' eggs. It was generally thought in the West of Scotland that a poultice of peeled onions, laid on the stomach, or underneath the armpits, would relieve one who had taken poison. Cogan, in his *Haven of Health*, says that for a cough onions should be roasted under hot embers and eaten with honey, and pepper and butter, morning and evening.†

Of the fame of vervain all old writers speak; and to carry it about on you was to secure you from the barking of dogs and the bites of snakes. To bind it to the head would cure headache. When it was gathered the gatherer was to say, according to a MS. of Elizabeth's reign,—

> "All-hale, thou holy herb, Vervin,
> Growing on the ground;
> In the Mount of Calvary
> There wast thou found;
> Thou helpest many a grief
> And stanchest many a wound.

---

* *Notes and Queries*, 5th S. vol. i. p. 505; Cockayne, vol. i. p. 119; Culpepper, p. 50; Floyer (*Touchstone of Medicine*, 1687) says the ashes of cabbage "are very caustick: the seed is bitter and acrid. The juyce cures warts."—vol. i. p. 213.

† *Domestic Annals of Scotland*, vol. iii. p. 55; Culpepper, p. 176; Napier, *Folk-Lore*, p. 127; Cogan, p. 59.

> In the name of sweet Jesus
> I take thee from the ground.
> O Lord, effect the same
> That I do now go about."

and also,—

> "In the name of God on Mount Olivet
> First I thee found;
> In the name of Jesus
> I pull thee from the ground."*

The universal cure for nettle-stings is to rub with the docken leaf and say,—

> "Out nettle,
> In dock,
> Dock shall have
> A new smock."

or,—

> "Nettle out, dock in,
> Dock remove the nettle-sting,"

or similar words. Dock-tea is sometimes recommended as a cure for boils. It is made from the root, well boiled, and is not of an agreeable flavour. Culpepper, two hundred years ago, said dock was strengthening to the liver, "yet such is the nicety of our times, (forsooth,") he adds, "that women will not put it in the pot because it makes the pottage black. Pride and ignorance (a couple of monsters in the creation) preferring nicety before health." St. Fabian's nettle is said to be a favourite remedy for consumption, and every book on folk-lore quotes the story of the mermaid of the Clyde who exclaimed when she beheld with regret the funeral of a young Glasgow maiden—

> "If they wad drink nettles in March,
> And eat muggins in May,
> Sae many braw maidens
> Wadna gang to clay."

---

* Cockayne, *Saxon Leechdoms*, vol. i. pp. 91, 93, 171; Harland and Wilkinson, *Lancashire Folk-Lore*, p. 76.

Katherine Oswald prescribed for the cure of "trymbling fevers" (ague), plucking a nettle by the root three successive mornings before sunrise. Tea made from young tops of nettles is a Derbyshire cure for nettle-rash.*

If peony were always carried, he who bore it need never feel insanity; or if a man were insane, to lay peony on him would soon restore him to health. A necklace made of beads turned from the root of the peony is used by West Sussex children to aid them in getting their teeth, and to prevent convulsions. Culpepper says peony is a herb of the sun, and under Leo. Physicians say male peony roots are the best, but Dr. Reason, he says, told him male peony was best for man, and female peony for women, and he desired to be judged by his brother, Dr. Experience. "The roots are held to be of more virtue than the seed; next, the flowers, and last of all, the leaves. The root of the male peony, fresh gathered, having been found by experience to cure the falling sickness, but the surest way is (besides hanging it about the neck, by which children have been cured) to take the root of the male peony washed clean, and stamped somewhat small, and laid to infuse in sack for twenty-four hours at the least; after strain it, and take it first and last, morning and evening, a good draft for sundry days together, before and after a full moon." "A mystical root, Baaras," Dalyell notes, "conjectured to be a species of peony, a noted expulsor, grew near Jerusalem, whence perhaps the repute of peony and its suspension from the neck of epileptic children." †

To the East both the ash and the mistletoe owe their almost sacred merits. Taking the last first we find that persons in Sweden who are afflicted with the falling sickness carry with them a knife, having a handle of oak mistletoe, to ward off

* *English Folk-Lore*, p. 172; Culpepper, pp. 87, 171; Dalyell (*Trial of Katharine Oswald*, 11 November, 1629, *Rec. Jus.*), p. 28; R. C. II. April, 1879.

† Cockayne, vol. i. p. 171; *Folk-Lore Record*, vol. i. p. 44; Culpepper, p. 186; Dalyell, *Darker Superstitions*, p. 612.

attacks. A piece of mistletoe hung round the neck would ward off other sicknesses. We have Culpepper's authority for saying it is excellent good for the grief of the sinew, itch, sores, and toothache, the biting of mad dogs and venomous beasts, and that it purgeth choler very gently.* Grimm notes that it was with a branch of mistletoe Baldur was killed,—" Ein kraut," he continues, "von dem des tod eines des grössten, geliebtesten götter abhing, muss für hochheilig erachtet worden sein, doch seine heiligkeit war wiederum deutschen und celtischen völkern gemein." † The *Kadeir Taliasin* says the mistletoe was one of the ingredients in the *awen a gwybodeu*, or water of inspiration, science, and immortality, which the goddess Ked prepared in her cauldron. Witches were thought to have no power to hurt those who bore mistletoe round their neck.‡ Sir Thomas Browne speaks of the virtues of mistletoe in cases of epilepsy.

To give a child ash sap, I have elsewhere noticed, was one of the first cares of a Scotch nurse, and sometimes weakly children were washed in dew from the leaves of the sacred tree. The sap tapped on certain days in spring is said to be drunk in Germany as a remedy for serpent bites. *The English Physician* has an explanation which was no doubt regarded as perfectly satisfactory. The saying that ash tree tops and leaves are good against the bites of serpents and vipers Culpepper supposes to have come from Gerard or Pliny, who both held that there is such antipathy between an adder and an ash tree that if an adder be compassed round with ash tree leaves it will sooner run through the fire than through the leaves. But this Culpepper does not believe. " The contrary," he says, " is truth, as both my eyes are witnesses." Apparently he tried the experiment, and found

---

* Kelly, *Curiosities*, p. 186 ; Culpepper, *English Physician*, p. 3.
† Grimm, *Deutsche Mythologie*, vol. ii. p. 1008.
‡ *Journal British Archæological Association*, vol. xxxiv. p. 484; Coles, *Art of Simpling* (1656), p. 67.

the adder to prefer the leaves to the fire. For sore ears the Saxon leeches said, take a green ashen staff, lay it in the fire, then take the juice that issues from it, put it on some wool, wring it into the ear, and stop the ear with the same wool. The wood of the ash cut at certain holy seasons was held to be incorruptible and to heal wounds. The spear of Achilles if it wounded could also cure if only the ashen shaft was applied to the wound.* " Rowan, ash, and red thread," a Scotch rhyme goes, " keep the devils frae their speed."† It was from the ash tree Iggdrasil that the gods formed man. Availing myself of Mr. Kelly's note on Iggdrasil and the Greek ash, I quote the following passage :—" The latter," he says, " was, like the former, a honey-dropping tree. Its name implies no less, for *melia* ash, and *meli, melit,* honey, have the same root, *mel,* which is found in many other words with the sense of sweet, pleasing, delightful. There was a positive as well as a mystic reason why the Greeks should give a name signifying sweetness, because the *Fraxinus ornus,* a species of ash indigenous in the South of Europe, yields manna from its slit bark. They may also have conceived that honey dropped from the earth as dew from the heavenly ash, for Theophrastus mentions a kind of honey which fell in that form from the air, and which was therefore called *aeromeli.* We now perceive the reason why the honey-giving nymphs of ash, and the honey-giving bees (melissai), were so assimilated in the minds of the Greeks that the nurses of the infant Zeus (Meliai) were called by them indifferently Meliat

---

* *English Physician Enlarged,* p. 21 ; Cockayne, vol. ii. p. 43 ; Kelly, pp. 147, 148, 152.

† *Choice Notes* (*Folk-Lore*), p. 24. The bay tree shared this power. "It is a tree of the sun, and under the celestial sign Leo, and resisteth witchcraft very potently, as also all the evils old Saturn can do to the body of man, and they are not a few ; for it is the speech of one, and I am mistaken if it were not Mizaldus, that neither witch nor devil, thunder nor lightning, will hurt a man in a place where a bay tree is."—Culpepper, p. 25.

and Melissai."* Martius says that ash wood is credited with healing wounds by its touch (Vulnera lignum fraxinum attactu sanare). Some, he continues, make a stick of the wood, when the sun and moon are in conjunction in Aries, by the mere touch of which stick any bleeding can be stopped.†

Armstrong, in his poem on the *Art of Preserving Health*, says,

> "Mark where the dry champaign
> Swells into cheerful hills; where Marjoram
> And *Thyme*, the love of bees, perfume the air,
> There bid thy roofs, high on the basking steep,
> Ascend; there light thy hospitable fires."

The correspondent who drew my attention to this passage observed that doubtless the air of the hills had more to do with their salubrity than the presence of the thyme and marjoram,‡ and it is not probable that the use Cornwall folk make of thyme occurred to the poet. A relation of mine was in the cottage of a wise woman at Penzance about two years ago, and found that she was still in the habit of prescribing in scrofulous cases grammar sows, sow-pigs, millepedes or woodlice, to be swallowed as a pill. According to the Penzance woman, the sufferer must himself secure his medicine, but she had a corner in her little garden where nothing was grown but mint and thyme, and there the sow-pigs were reared. As a concession to modern feelings, patients are now allowed to wear this disagreeable medicine in a little bag round the neck, if they shrink from the heroic remedy of swallowing it.§

---

* *Indo-European Tradition*, p. 144.
† Martius, p. 32.
‡ G. L. A. (Wimbledon), 17 January, 1879.
§ Miss M. L. B. 17 October, 1878. "In the Eastern Counties they are called *old-sows* and sow-bugs, and in other parts St. Anthony's hogs. Their Latin name is *porcellio scaber*. The Welsh have several names for this insect,— *gwrach-y-coed*, *i.e.* the withered old woman of the wood; *gwrach-y-lludw*;

DOMESTIC FOLK-MEDICINE. 199

A poisonous bean, Esëre, is used by the natives of Calabar when an ulcer appears on the foot. One or two beans are laid on the sore, because whatever witch may have had power to cause the ulcer she can have no power to continue her evil work when the beans are there, for her influence cannot penetrate them.* Black bean tree is a cure for nettlerush in Berkshire.

Silver weed if steeped in butter-milk is said to remove freckles and brownness. *Cork* is thought to have the power of keeping off cramp if placed between the bed and mattress, or between the sheets. This is a Lincolnshire recipe. Sometimes cork garters are made by sewing together thin pieces of cork between two sick ribbons.† The excrescence found on a briar sore, and called *Robin Redbreast's cushion*, is said in Sussex to be the finest thing known for whooping-cough.‡ *Peas* are thought in Germany good for all complaints, but particularly wounds and bruises; children suffering from measles should be washed in water in which peas have been boiled. The leaves of the *peach* were, according to the *Three Hundred Receipts* of 1724, to be applied when children suffered from worms. Culpepper says, "Lady Venus owns this tree." The juice of the stalk of the *dandelion* is used in Derbyshire to cure warts. A Donegal wise woman gives her patient nine leaves of dandelion, or heart fever grass, as she calls it, and directs him to eat three leaves

gwrach-y-twed. Gwrach means a withered old woman, so also does *grammar*; so that grammar is but an English equivalent of *gwrach*. Other Welsh names are mochyn-y-coed, *i.e.* the little pig of the wood; and tyrchyn llwyd, *i.e.* the little grey hog."—W. N., *Cornishman*, 17 October, 1878.

* *Christian Express* (Lovedale, South Africa), Oct. 1878, p. 11; R. C. H. 25 April, 1879.

† Pratt, *Wild Flowers*, vol. ii. p. 32.

‡ *Folk-Lore Record*, vol. i. p. 38. "I recollect a growth of this kind of unusual size being given to a little girl, who had whooping-cough, as a plaything. On seeing it the nurse exclaimed, 'I am glad to see that. I have been wishing for one for several days to hang round Miss Mary's neck.'"

on three successive mornings. She gathers the dandelion herself.*

Eyebright (*Euphrasia*) made into powder, and then into an electuary with sugar, "hath," says Culpepper, "powerful effect to help and restore the sight decayed through age, and Arnoldus de villa nova saith, it hath restored sight to them that have been blind a long time before."† It was thus the Archangel Michael opened Adam's eyes,

> " Michael from Adam's eyes the film removed
> Which that false fruit, which promised clearer sight
> Had bred ; then purged with euphrasy and rue
> The visual nerve for he had much to see."

Shenstone in his *Schoolmistress* says,

> " Euphrasy may not be left unsung,
> That gives dim eyes to wander leagues around."

The Tyrolese agree with Milton as to the merits of rue, saying that it confers fine vision, and used with agrimony, it is prescribed in Posen for serpent bites. In England, six ounces of rue, cleaned picked and bruised, boiled in ale, with certain quantities of garlic, treacle, and scraped tin in a clean covered pot, over a gentle fire, has been recommended for the bite of a mad dog. When the compound was strained, eight or nine spoonfuls of it were to be given to the man or woman three mornings fasting, within nine days of the bite. Some of the ingredients might, when convenient, be with advantage bound on the wound.‡

* Kelly, pp. 299, 300; *Three Hundred Receipts*, p. 113 ; *English Physician Enlarged*, p. 180; R. C. H. 25 April, 1879; "Fairy Superstitions in Donegal," *University Mag.* August 1879, p. 217.

† *English Physician Enlarged*, p. 97. " Ignored by the faculty, the Herbal became the guide of the quack ; and in Culpepper's famous Herbal it had become a fit companion for the Astrological Almanac. This was the dotage of that ancient partnership between Botany and Medicine which in Dioscorides was young and sound."—Earle, *English Plant Names*, p. xxviii.

‡ Conway, *Demonology*, vol. ii. p. 324 ; R. S. H. April, 1879.

The celebrity of mugwort (*artemisia vulgaris*) is great.
Cockayne gives a poem descriptive of this eldest of worts:

"Thou hast might for three
And against thirty,
For venom availest
For plying vile things."

The *Herbarium Apuleii* says, mugwort puts away madness, and in whatever house it is no evil crafts can have power, and evil eyes will be turned away.* The roots used to be collected on St. John's day.

A poultice made of rotten apple is applied in Lincolnshire to cure eyes affected by rheumatism or weakness; it is in the commonest possible use. A charm for the bite of a mad dog, communicated by Professor Marecco, was to be written on an apple, or a piece of fine white bread. It begins, "O King of Glory, come in peace."†

Crowsfoot is mentioned as used for the cure of a kenning, or keming, white spot on the eye.‡ In use it is to be accompanied by a muttered incantation. Yarrow worn in a little bag upon the stomach was the secret against agues of a great lord, who himself confided this to Boyle. The lord was very curious of receipts, and would sometimes pay highly for them, and a very famous physician of Boyle's acquaintance informed him that the yarrow had been used with strange success.§ Common fumitory, which John Clare says "superstition holds to Fame," was used when gathered in wedding hours, and boiled in water, milk, and whey, as a wash for the complexion of rustic maids. Amaranth,

"which once
In Paradise, fast by the tree of life,
Began to bloom."

---

* Cockayne, vol. iii. p. 30 ; vol. i. p. 103.
† Rev. G. S. S. 24 October, 1878 ; Henderson, *Folk-Lore of the Northern Counties*, p. 179.
‡ Polwhele, *Traditions and Recollections*, vol. ii. p. 607.
§ Boyle, *Some Considerations, &c.* vol. i. p. 211.

has medicinal merits, for its flowers are said to stop bleeding at the nose, or of a wound.

A broth of tripe boiled in water, with spices and vegetables, was considered, Scarron says, a remedy against rheumatism. Fuller's teazle (*dipsacus fullonum*) is thought, in some parts of England, a certain remedy for ague. Leaves of ivy steeped in water for a day and a night were thought to cure sore and smarting eyes. Cups made from ivy were recommended for use in cases of spleen, or of whooping-cough. "Cato saith, That wine put into such a cup will soak through it, by reason of the antipathy that is between them."* Laurel was deemed a preservative against epilepsy, and thence an antidote to madness. Fumigating byres with juniper is supposed to ward off disease in Aberdeenshire, and the *English Physician* says of juniper, "this admirable solar shrub is scarcely to be paralleled for his virtues." †

Kolb, who became one of the first "wonder doctors" of the Tyrol, when he was called to assist any bewitched person, made exactly at midnight the smoke of five different sorts of herbs, and while they were burning the bewitched was gently beaten with a martyr-thorn birch, which had to be got the same night. This beating the patient with thorn was thought to be really beating the hag who had caused the evil.‡ A Derbyshire cure for chilblains is to thrash them with holly.

To bite the first seen fern that appears in spring off by the ground is said, in Cornwall and elsewhere, to cure toothache, and to prevent its return during the remainder of the year; as to fever, "eine art angang ist es, dass die drei ersten korn oder schlehblüthen, deren man im jahr ansichtig wird, heilmittel wider das fieber abgeben." § The first blackberry seen will, Cornish

---

* Scarron, *Adieu au Marais et à la Place Royal*, complete works, vol. iv. p. 32 ; *English Folk-Lore*, pp. 21, 22 ; Culpepper, p. 135.

† Dalyell, p. 139 ; Culpepper, p. 136.

‡ Comtesse von Günther, *Tales and Legends of the Tyrol*, pp. 105-106.

§ Grimm, *Deutsche Mythologie*, vol. ii. p. 978.

people say, banish warts. The bracken, witches are said to detest, because it bears on its root the letter C, the initial of the holy name.* The root of the yellow *iris*, chopped up and chewed, is said to be an Argyleshire cure for toothache. *Broom* tree is a cure for dropsy in Derbyshire. For chilblains, sore eyes, and chapped hands, the juice of leek squeezed out and mixed with cream is said to be a cure. To escape a curtain lecture, or, as the Saxon more rudely puts it, "against a woman's chatter," one should taste at night, fasting, a root of radish, and chatter will not be able to harm him.† To cure a woman of dumbness, on the other hand, we have the authority of one of the *C. Mery Talys* that an aspen leaf is the proper thing to put under her tongue.‡

* "A friend suggests, however, that the letter intended is not the English C but the Greek χ, the initial letter of the word χριστος, which really resembles very closely the marks in the root of the bracken, or *Pteris aquilina*."—Henderson, p. 226. "For thigh aches (sciatica) smoke the thighs thoroughly with fern."—Cockayne, vol. ii. p. 65.
† Cockayne, vol. ii. p. 343.
‡ *A. C. Mery Talys*, p. 87 (*Shakespeare Jest Books*).

CHAPTER XIII.

THE PLACE OF FOLK-MEDICINE IN THE STUDY OF CIVILISATION.

E have now discussed the theories of Folk-Medicine in some detail. Beginning with primitive conceptions of the origin of diseases and death, we saw how naturally a theory of Transference of Disease might arise, and what influence has been exercised by Association of Ideas—exemplified, in one way, in a doctrine of Sympathy, and in another in Symbolic new birth. The curious group of myths which have collected around the persons of our Lord and the Saints was then noticed. Connected quite as much with this Christian mythology—I trust I shall not be misunderstood in using this term—as with pre-Christian mythology there is an important set of factors, regarded here under the names of Colour, Number, and Influence of the Sun and Moon. In personal cures we have perhaps examples of personal fetish—occasionally illustrations of adapted theology; cures associated with animals, or the habits of animals, serve to remind us of the survival of belief in animal-fetishes in modern societies; and in collecting and comparing Magic writings and notes on rings, and those miscellaneous charms (which have been indicated as presently falling under a general title of "Domestic Folk-Medicine"), materials have been provided for future conjecture as to the meaning which is to be attached to many beliefs and superstitions as yet but roughly classable.

I cannot but be conscious that in suggesting as the three

primitive explanations of disease,—(1) the anger of an offended external spirit; (2) the supernatural powers of a human enemy; and (3) the displeasure of the dead, and especially in placing these suggestions in the above order,—I may seem to have ignored the conclusions to which Mr. Spencer believes he can point as the result of study of primitive man. Mr. Spencer, using the phrase ancestor-worship in its broadest sense as comprehending all worship of the dead, be they of the same blood or not, concludes that ancestor-worship is the root of every religion (*The Data of Sociology*, p. 440). He says " it becomes manifest that setting out with the wondering double which the dream suggests; passing to the double that goes away at death; advancing from this ghost, at first supposed to have but a transitory second life, to ghosts which exist permanently and therefore accumulate,—the primitive man is led gradually to people surrounding space with supernatural beings which inevitably become in his mind causal agents for everything unfamiliar." (*Ibid.* p. 450.) Mr. Spencer finds then that, generally, all primitive theories attribute disease and death to the spirits of the dead.

With this theory I must disagree. The order of explanations may not, taking humanity as a whole, be the same everywhere,—although in all probability it is generally the same,—and I have expressly stated my doubts if we can rank one theory above another in importance, or assign to this or that greater or less influence; but, so far as all our knowledge goes at present, I cannot accept Mr. Spencer's arguments as convincing, so far as Folk-Medicine is concerned. There is abundant proof of the fear of the dead, of their worship, of their propitiation, of belief in their malice and their love; but I do not think that any dogmatic assertion can be safely made that from fear of dreams or of disembodied spirits arose all primitive man's theories of disease and death; much less, then, his apprehension of a Supreme Power, or, speaking generally, his religion.

Mr. Spencer is very desirous that we should recollect how many difficulties present themselves when we endeavour to place ourselves in the position of totally uneducated, untrained, almost unknowing beings; and it is certainly well, from time to time, to point out the great care which is necessary in framing imaginary yet rational theories for primitive man. In all Mr. Spencer advances on this point every student of civilisation will agree with him. Too great caution is impossible. To a great extent Mr. Spencer is entitled to credit for analysing and classifying savage beliefs in a spirit of the most impartial kind. At the same time, without expressing any opinion upon Mr. Spencer's theory of religion, or the Evolutionist arguments with which he builds up his Castle Doubting, I am unable to regard his first step, his initial premises, as either actually or possibly accurate.

Primitive man presents himself to us in two aspects. Mentally he is a child, physically he is a hardy savage; for, as the doctrine of the survival of the fittest may here be rigidly and accurately applied, it is clear that under pristine conditions of life only the most healthy could attain manhood. Primitive man is a healthy animal, with a brain capable of development. It is necessary to bear in mind these two aspects, if we are to judge accurately of man's primitive conceptions of things. If we omit either the hardihood of the body or the infancy of the mind we are not likely to escape hasty and erroneous conclusions.

What, then, does this twofold aspect teach regarding such a theory of mental evolution as that of Mr. Spencer? First of all, that we must be cautious what physical ailments we ascribe to man. Here is a healthy savage, what are likely to be the conditions pressed upon him. Hunger and repletion, no doubt; but what else? apoplexy and epilepsy, delirium, insanity? Surely not. Even among ourselves these are comparatively rare experiences. I grant that the more rare the more likely would they be to make strong suggestive impressions upon the mind of primitive man, but I demur to any doctrine that man's earliest conceptions were in the least degree likely to be materially due to those disorders. Greatly they may have modified, or even entirely altered, his first conceptions, but the savage, primarily and necessarily healthy, was neither apoplectic nor epileptic. I argue, as does Mr. Spencer, from the presumed state of man's nature when intellect dawned.

Primitive man again has a mind like a child's mind—that is to say, he has a mind like a looking-glass, which reflects all and retains nothing. It will show the image of this or that, but remove the object and its image vanishes. Mr. Spencer himself cites instances of this state of mind in savage communities. It is illustrated by Mr. Oldfield's difficulties with the Australians. If he asked a question they immediately assented. A native brought him some specimens of a species of eucalyptus: " Being desirous of ascertaining the habit of the plant, I asked, 'A tall tree?' to which his ready answer was in the affirmative. Not feeling quite satisfied I again demanded, 'A low bush?' to which 'Yes' was also the response." The Damaras have great difficulty in counting beyond five, because no other hand remains to secure the units already counted. Many instances of primitive man's feeble grasp of thought, as illustrated in such people, as may be presumed approximately to represent him might be collected.* I shall assume, therefore, that admittedly man, so far as we can learn from his history as written in himself, is mentally fairly represented by a very young civilised child.

The conclusions to which Mr. Spencer would point, then, are that to this strong, childlike savage the first explanation of disease, of death, and the suggestion of higher powers and religion, are due to dreams and epileptic fits. The healthy savage delays all conjectures about life or death till he sees his

* See Lubbock, *Origin of Civilization*, pp. 8, 9; Spencer, *Data of Sociology*, pp. 94 *et seq.*

brother writhe in convulsions; he thinks of nothing till he has pondered over the dreams, which he cannot disassociate from reality, caused by hunger or overfeeding. These are a couple of untenable propositions. The case of the child is itself an illustration of the error. Take a child of three years old that can run, and play, and speak, ask it about its dreams, draw any picture you like of what it may have seen, get its brothers of six or seven to ask questions in their own way, and to all the reply will be alike indicative of the mind of primitive man—either there will be a blank denial of dreams and all such things, or a ready "Yes" to suggestions the most preposterous. On the other hand, show such a child a picture, and he will pick out the image which he has learnt to associate with the living dog by his side; better still, play music to him, sing to him, and he from day to day will have stronger and truer recollections of every rhythm and every tune.

Did primitive man, living in nature, on Nature's purest, roughest products, ignore altogether his world of wind, sea, and sky, and find the first wakening of his dormant mind in dreams and illnesses? I do not, of course, say that a child may not have very real dreams which he thinks about. He may believe them to be so real that he can form no idea of their non-reality. This is quite conceivable; all the same, he does not betray in his daily play indications of a life apart from that of his nursery. His dream-life may be the very counterpart of his waking-life, but it does not exercise over him the effect which the dream-life of many modern savage tribes exercises over them. This may be, because, before the dream-interpretation-faculty is properly conceived, the mind of the civilised child is distracted to other things. But here is the admission that a dream-interpretation-faculty takes time to develop—is, then, during all the time of development, primitive man to be blind and insensible to external nature, and to the influence of his brother man? I claim, therefore, that the mythologist, to use Mr. Spencer's term, far more accurately grasps the ideas and feelings of the semi-civilised than does the Spencerean thinker. Mr. Spencer misses the first step; if that be allowed, then, indeed, one may do what he pleases in adjusting the data of sociology. No thinker or writer of the present age can form a true, that is an absolutely true, idea of primitive man from such tribes and peoples as have so far lagged behind in the race of life that they represent to us conditions of existence which we call prehistoric, so far as the history of mankind at large is concerned. Mr. Spencer assumes that we can judge of the past by the present in the very particulars which others might think the most liable to alteration, possibly to mental variations corresponding with the physical, or at least social inferiority—not impossibly degradation—of the peoples among whom they are now found. Professor Max Müller has said, "the more we go back, the more we examine the earliest germs of every religion, the purer, I believe, we shall find the conceptions of the Deity." Mr. Spencer regards this assertion as due to a perversion of thought, caused by looking at facts in the wrong order. I am not called upon here to examine the primitive conceptions of God, but I have no doubt, speaking from my own study of the data of sociology as embodied in folk-medicine (but not confined to this data alone), that the primary intuition of man was conception of external nature power. I put this very broadly, for I think that if primitive man saw his brother struck by lightning he believed his fall was due to some cause, similar to that which made his brother fall if he were struck, or if a branch felled him. The cause was external; it might be invisible; he did not reason; he did not ask, What relation has this external force which made my brother fall to me and to him? Like a child, he received the impression of something beyond himself—like himself in the results which followed —unlike himself in being invisible.

Mr. Spencer finds an argument against Nature, recognition in the fact that "the familiar Sun excites in the child no awe whatever." "Recalling his boyhood," continues he, "no one can recall any feeling of fear drawn out by this most striking object in Nature, or any sign of such feeling in his companions. Again, what peasant or what servant-girl betrays the slightest reverence for the Sun? Gazed at occasionally, admired, perhaps, when setting, it is regarded without even a tinge of the sentiment called worship." &c.*

This is an unfortunate illustration, for if there is one particular respect in which the modern child greatly differs from the primitive man it is in the different conditions of his daily life. Mentally the conceptions of the one may justifiably be taken to illustrate those of the other. In ways of life they are very different. When, for example, does the civilised child see the Sun either rise or set? To what extent again is he dependent upon its warmth? What does winter mean more than nursery fires? What does night mean save bed-time? There is no analogy whatever between the conditions of life of the civilised child and the savage. The savage knows that when that distant shining ball appears, there is light; when it apparently has slid or climbed across the sky there is no light, *i.e.*, dark. This is surely the most primitive of conceptions. The savage does not theorise about this, nor build up myths; he receives the facts of light and darkness, but in his reception of those facts is the unconscious exercise of thought, far anterior surely to concern about his dreams (only themselves, as a rule, to come when the sun is gone), far more ancient than speculations as to the nervous convulsions of friend or foe. It is not necessary to our argument to think of the savage as given to "imaginative fictions." It would rather seem as if the need of an assumption of "imaginative fictions" would be required in the arguments of those who, as it were, put their hand over the first lines of the History of Culture, and begin with the second paragraph. Certainly the savage is characterised by lack of imagination,

* *Data of Sociology*, Appendix B, p. t.

but his imagination, when it is touched, is most truly touched by facts which appeal suggestively to him. I am far from denying the great importance attached by men, apparently representative of primitive man, to dreams, ghosts or spirits of the dead. I have recognised this as the third primitive theory of the origin of disease and death, but so far as the real primitive man is concerned, I conjecture, even putting altogether out of account the possibilities of peculiar spiritual revelation—inconceivable to us now, if confined to the leaden facts of Mr. Spencer—that primitive man was influenced, first of all, by either the facts of external animate and inanimate nature (not human), the facts of human life, as seen in the coeval actions of his healthy brothers, the one acting and re-acting, modifying, transforming, the other from time to time, and as the capacities, the surroundings, the health, the circumstances of individual man varied. After this I admit the importance of the ghost theory fully, and the possibility of this theory so affecting the first conceptions, that any one arguing from mere latter facts, and ignoring the necessary conditions of the actual primitive man's life, might very well assume the pure nature, and the simple fellow-man influences to be unreal and imaginary. They are not, however, necessarily unreal or untrue, because they cannot now be completely proved by the arguments Mr. Spencer would alone employ.

For these reasons I adhere to my first classification of the theories of the origin of disease and death which I believe to have affected primitive man. The data given on an earlier page need not here be repeated, but I would point out, as a necessary warning, that such data as have been collected in the case of the first two theories are not relied upon as proving any conclusion advanced here. Even if they were entirely satisfactory as evidence of a state of society similar to that of primitive man, which might furnish safe evidence as to his mental conceptions,

I would not ground any arguments upon them.* We may entirely transcend the mere facts of bricks and stones when we visit a great mansion, but we may be sure that they are there. We can safely assume that a great river is fed by many tributaries, although we only see it widening into an ocean. In a word, we need not, must not, forego assumptions in reason when we examine facts.

In the above remarks I refer to Mr. Spencer's system of philosophy only in so far as it seems to me inconsistent with a correct study of Folk-Medicine, and of the place of Folk-Medicine in the history of civilisation.

Turning to Folk-Medicine itself,—in the chapters which precede I have endeavoured to show the interest and importance which attaches to study of folk-medicine. Charms, spells, and amulets, trifling and unimportant in themselves and in reference to modern medicine, take an altogether different aspect when viewed together as a whole, in illustration of that mental progress of society which is more correctly indicated by the word "culture" than by "civilisation." They cease to be merely melancholy or ludicrous facts, absurd and humiliating; they are really far more than this, they are like leafless trees in winter, naked and unsheltering, but still useful in pointing out the way which the snow has concealed. By their help we recover the road before the night conceals all.

It is not surprising that the collection of scraps of superstitious lore should have been ridiculed. It is more wonder-

* Even Mr. Spencer does not seem to regard primitive man as accurately represented by the peoples upon whose superstitions and beliefs he grounds his theory:—" To determine what conceptions are truly primitive, would be easy if we had accounts of truly primitive men. But there are sundry reasons for suspecting that existing men of the lowest types, forming social groups of the simplest kinds, do not exemplify men as they originally were. Probably most of them, if not all of them, had ancestors in higher states; and among their beliefs remain some which were evolved during those higher states . . . It is quite possible, and, I believe, highly probable, that retrogression has been as frequent as progression."—*Data of Sociology*, p. 106.

ful that so much ancient lore remains imbedded in the common speech and thought of every-day life. It is remarkable that in the present day we should so often be able to trace a custom or a saying to times of remote antiquity. The conclusion to which the possibility of tracing our culture back to early days seems to point is, that intellectually as well as physically we may still approximately study the past in the present. We know that in Scotland cave-life is still to be found at Wick Bay, and that beehive houses are still inhabited in the Hebrides ; and in the same way we know from the collections of folk-lore which have of late been made, that there are men and women living in this year in our civilised communities whose reasoning power on some subjects has never progressed beyond limits which we find adequately indicated in the tales of barbarous or semi-barbarous (but not necessarily primitive) tribes. Mental training and civilisation alike travel irregularly; in some cases rapidly, in others very slowly. Thus there is the possibility in civilisation of the luxury of all the world in London, and the most primitive barbarity in the north of Scotland ; and in culture there is the possibility of hundreds and thousands of educated brains co-existing with men whose thinking powers are still dormant. But the two cases of civilisation and culture are not quite parallel. There is one great difference. We should not expect to find modern cave-dwellings on any part of the Thames banks, but we may find in one house, under one roof, a student of the most recent science, and a boor who still hunts for the fern which is to make him invisible, and who respectfully salutes a magpie. The better-educated portion of the world is naturally the authority as to the less educated portion ; this, in the nature of things, must always be ; none the less, the judgment under those circumstances to be pronounced we may be justified in regarding as one-sided. It is here, then, that one instance of the value of the study of folk-lore appears. The current thoughts of the real body of the people are by it ascertained ; we learn by it the nature of the foundation on which conjectures and hypotheses are based. We may get no clear statement of this or that belief; we are like school-boys who do not write essays in their first year, but begin by learning signs, then combine signs into words, and then words into sentences. To learn the signs is the first and most important part of the task; this learned, all else will follow in due course. Thus, to collect the proverbs, sayings, the superstitions of any town or country people is the first task; when so much progress has been made a broader view can be taken of all which those represent. Finally, two advantages result from the inquiry—in the first place, there is something learnt by the study of the living present of what was regarded as the dead past, the tables are turned for the moment upon the better-educated portion of the community, and we see the nation at large as it is, not as it appears to a class of peculiar education and training; in the second place, we can look back upon the intellectual history of our people with some certainty that that history is not entirely unreadable.

To collect odd phrases and scraps of folk-lore and string them together for the benefit of the curious is not to investigate folk-lore; it is rather to bring ill-deserved ridicule upon a study which has not for its object the pastime of a leisure hour, but the investigation of the greatest problem which man can solve — the growth of his mental faculties. If students of folk-lore had any less end in view they could not ask for their pursuit serious consideration; and they would deserve neither sympathy nor assistance in their work. It is as a serious contribution to the history of man's life in this world from the dawn of his intellectual being that each work based on investigation of primitive habits and primitive phases of thought must be regarded. It does not appear to be vain to believe that by such inquiry there is more probability of ultimate knowledge of this difficult subject being reached, than by almost any other way, if it is possible, as I believe it is, to go back by the aid of folk-lore to ages, and, what is of more importance, to stages of life and thought which can otherwise in no way be reached. Bit by bit very slowly the work will go on; and it is as a small contribution to this work that the notes of which this book is composed have been collected.

In one respect this volume may be said to depart somewhat widely from the lines indicated by the three masters of research in the field of sociological inquiry,—Mr. Spencer, Dr. Tylor, and Sir John Lubbock. I have drawn more examples of the various branches of folk-medicine from the folk-lore of our own country than from that of foreign and savage lands. I quite admit that even the most ignorant countryman in the British Isles is very far in advance of primitive man; he has wants, he has luxuries, he has desires, he has ambitions which only become realizable by the human race after very long preliminary training. But in a way which seems to me very remarkable many of our countrymen are *in* civilization but not *of* it. So far as their social life is concerned, so far as their life is dependent upon or united with the life of others, they are representative and typical only of their class of modern society. But this is only one aspect of their life. So far as their mental position is not dependent upon habits forced from without they are beyond the sphere of modern thoughts. For example, a man such as I refer to may go to church all his life as his fathers did, and hear nothing save the parson "a bummin' awaay loike a buzzard-clock." He will vote for church and state, and drift with the stream of external things which came he knows not whence and goes he knows not where. Mentally he has two conceptions. It is difficult to make clear the vast depth between the notions which he has simply received, as water is received by an empty vessel, and the notions which are of his own investigation, laboured out as a savage burns out his canoe from a tree trunk. The one stage is illustrated by the same Northern Farmer:—

"I niver know'd whot a meän'd but I thawt a' ad summat to saäy,
An' I thawt a said a owt to 'a snid an' I coom'd awaäy."

He receives the external opinion of things; he conforms to custom with its rule stronger than iron; like the Thibetan he turns his wheel of prayer, and, when he has done what he thinks custom requires him to do, he comes away. The other stage, that of laboured thought, is illustrated by the country explanations of current things in a matter-of-fact way; as that the dancing light of muddy swamps is borne by a radiant something, by-and-bye personalized and named Will o' the Wisp. If there is a light, something must carry it; as it moves, it must be a person who carries it.

A high degree of comparative culture is seen to be compatible with the simple uninquiring, unmeaning receptiveness of the lowest races of men. The process which results in the ultimate survival of the fittest goes on more slowly now than ever before. It must be borne in mind also that one stunted human plant exercises incalculably more influence upon his species than any analogy from vegetable life can illustrate. Thus with the survival of incomplete forms of thought, of aberrated minds, of stunted mental trees, we have also to consider the effect of their human influence, for only to the observer can the peculiar incapacity of mind make itself apparent. We have all seen blind men whose pride or whose sensitiveness had taught them so well to simulate the ways of seeing men, that, had we not known, we could scarcely have told that they saw no sun, and read no book; in the same way there are hundreds, there have been thousands, of our own countrymen whose mental incapacity it is almost impossible to detect. It could not be detected by their habits, by their accustomed forms of life, by the food they ate, by their votes, by their church-going, but we can tell it by their tales, by their superstitions, by their proverbs, and by their charms.

It is one of the natural results, fortunate or unfortunate from the venue of the bystander, of thus working backwards, that as

FOLK-MEDICINE IN THE STUDY OF CIVILISATION. 217

we work we disinter facts which differ as much in their use and in their value as do gold and silver from lead and tin. Here we may come across a detail which is absent from a very ancient myth where we would have expected to find it, there we have an incident which illustrates the development of modern fact into modern fable. Thus there are two processes continually before us. On the one hand we accumulate links of that great chain which leads us from Piccadilly to the Garden of Eden, and on the other we see the development of new lines of thought as yet more in the domain of the politician than in that of the student of culture, although when comprehensively regarded they are of course matters for the same study. In one word we see both how the nations grew, and how a nation grows.

This then brings into view another aspect of the study of the history of civilisation. It is not only to amuse the curious I have said that culture is to be studied. To this I would add, neither is it alone for the edification of historians of mankind that stores of facts are to be laboriously accumulated, assorted, and described. It would be, after all, but a trifling work to provide merely a record of man's progress in life, work, and thought, if nothing were to be learnt from it in the future. Culture, rightly studied, must not only be a beacon which tells of cliffs and sands safely passed but also an indication of the safe " water-lane " which lies before the watching sailor. It is sometimes objected to archæology that its tendency is not to advance but to retard, that the objects on which it lavishes time, care, and money are of so little value to a working-day world that time, care, and money have alike all been wasted,—those boxes of precious ointment might have been sold and given to the poor; as it is, they are spilt upon the ground, neither to the profit of the soil nor the real benefit of the lavisher.

To this there is one short and speedy answer. Let it be admitted that more than once erudition and wealth have been frittered away on subjects which, if not entirely unworthy, were at least comparatively unimportant either to man's mental or man's physical well-being. There remains, however, an important residuum, and, apart altogether from the mere benefit to history and art of archæological research, there have been again and again many positive advantages of which the world would otherwise have been ignorant. To what do we owe the Renaissance of Italy and southern Europe,—to what in our own day do we owe the Gothic revival,—to what do we owe the hundred arts which make our life of to-day more beautiful to those who have leisure and wealth, and more varied—if not more happy—to the unfortunate poor, than has been any previous age in the world's history? Without question, the answer to be returned must surely be that all this is owing in very great measure to intelligent study of the things of the past,—and intelligent study of the things of the past is archæology.

For the archæology of the mind we may claim much the same arguments, while we admit a sensible distinction and difference.

Few things are more significant of the strange halts and pauses which mentally a people makes than to note how superstition springs up in the very midst of modern education. The same sun which encourages the wheat gives the tares fresh vigour. We all know how much the Evil Eye is feared; how much, particularly in the east, a mother dreads to be too effusively congratulated on the beauty of her child,—how great in all primitive communities is the tendency to deprecate too much praise, too much gratification, lest ill-luck should follow—the avenger of good fortune. By-and-bye, a power in actually inducing evil is believed to be specially settled in particular persons, who are avoided, and feared, and propitiated like inferior deities. Their glance is a curse, their presence is a cloud. Their evil influence is warded off by mystic signs and amulets. Now the belief in the Jettatura, every one knows, still exists in many forms, and in many countries.

To take another example which this indeed suggests. From

personal evil influence, evil influence at last attaches to things. Objects blessed or cursed by witches, pins, animals, food, all may be cause of evil. Their very presence, associated in the past with death or disgrace, may become ominous of dismay and terror in the present. Of this we have an example in such a belief as this, that it is unlucky to keep black-edged note paper in a house. It is clear what this means. Black-edged note paper is used when death is in a house, and then only. Hence, is not to keep it in a house almost as though one felt the dread shadow; then, if this is felt, is it not indeed present? But this must be a very modern superstition. Mourning note-paper is only of modern introduction. How strangely the mysterious past rules the utilitarian present.

Again, it is matter of common report in the daily newspapers, that burglars are very often, if not always, found to have a piece of coal in their pocket. Why should this be used? Surely a modern ruffian, who knows something of dynamite and nitro-glycerine, and is better acquainted with the use of fire-arms than most of those who either hunt him, or are assailed by him, cannot depend upon an amulet. Yet this seems certain. I do not know that coal has any folk-lore mystery, but I would hazard the suggestion that its colour may suggest, very dimly and remotely, to the burglar-mind, remote shadowy tales of invisibility. It is a curious physchological study in two ways, first, how the burglar comes to think of an amulet, and what he thinks it is or can do; and second, the burglar imagination, which throws a glamour of Asian romance over a chip of coal stolen from a passing cart.

But what place can Folk-Medicine claim in the great book of culture? This question cannot but occur over and over again to those who have examined charms, spells, and amulets. We know that Mr. Spencer builds upon what he regards as primary foundations of thought all his philosophy. I have already stated my objections to his conclusion. I do not differ from him, however, regarding the importance of sociology, and it is as a contribution to the history of the culture of societies that this book has been written. A separate theory of Folk-Medicine is impossible, for Folk-Medicine has been built up out of very strange and varied materials; but it is perhaps not altogether vain to hope that illustrations of man's intellectual history will be found by study of collections of classified facts, and that the investigation of spells and amulets, of superstitions and witcheries, may not be unworthy of systematic analysis.

BOOKS OF REFERENCE.

Anthropological Institute, Journal of
Antiquary, the (magazine)
Aubrey, John, Remaines of Gentilisme and Judaisme, ed. by Jas. Britten, 1881

Birch, W. de Gray, On Two Anglo-Saxon MSS. in the British Museum, 1876
Blumler, M. F., Amuletorum Historia, Magdeburg. 1710
Boyle, Some Considerations touching the Usefulness of Experimental Philosophy, 2nd ed. 1664
Brand, John, Description of Orkney, 703
——— Popular Antiquities, 1877 ed.
British Archaeological Association, Transactions of
Brown, Sir Thomas, Pseudodoxia Epidemica, 4th ed. 1658
Burton, Anatomy of Melancholy
Busk, Miss, Valleys of Tirol, 1874

Cameron, Across Africa
Catlin, Letters and Notes on North American Indians, 2 vols.
Chambers, Domestic Annals of Scotland, 3 vols.
——— Popular Rhymes of Scotland
Choice Notes, Folk-Lore, 1859
Christian Express, Lovedale, South Africa
Cockayne, Rev. O., Saxon Leechdoms, &c. 3 vols. 1864
Cogan, Haven of Health
Conrad, Elias, Disputatio Physica exhibens i. Doctrinam de Magia; ii. Thearemata Miscellanea, 1661
Contemporary Review, Oct. 1875

Conway, M.D., Demonology and Devil-Lore, 2 vols.
Croker, T. Crofton, Killarney Legends, 1879 ed.
Culpepper, Nich., The English Physician enlarged, 1684

Dalyell, John Graham, The Darker Superstitions of Scotland, 1835
Dennys, N. B., The Folk-Lore of China and its affinities with that of the Aryan and Semitic Races, 1876
Derbyshire Gatherer
Digby, Sir Kenelm, A Late Discourse made in a Solemn Assembly of Nobles and learned men at Montpellier in France, touching the cure of wounds by the powder of sympathy, &c. 3rd ed. 1660
D'Iharace, Erreurs populaires sur le Médecine, 1783
Dorman, R. M., The Origin of Primitive Superstitions, 1881
Dyer, Rev. T. F. Thiselton, English Folk-Lore, 1878

Earle, John, English Plant Names. 1880

Floyer, Touchstone of Medicine, 2 vols., 1687
Folk-Lore Journal, South African, vol. i.
Folk-Lore Record, vols. i. ii. iii. iv. (1878, 1879, 1880, 1881)
Giles, H. A., Strange Stories from a Chinese Studio, 2 vols. 1880
Gill, Myths and Songs from the South Pacific
Gould, Rev. S. Baring, Life of Rev. R. S. Hawker

SELECTED BOOKS OF REFERENCE.

Curious Myths of the Middle Ages, 1877
Gregor, Rev. Walter, Folk-Lore of the North-East of Scotland, 1881
Grimm, Jacob, Deutsche Mythologie Vierte ausgabe besorgt von Elard Hugo Meyer, 3 vols. i. (1875), ii. (1877). iii. (1878). *See* Stallybrass
Grohman, Tyrol and the Tyrolese
Günther, Countesse A. von, Tales and Legends of the Tyrol, 1874

Harland, John, and Wilkinson, T. T., Lancashire Folk-Lore, 1867
Harrison, Description of England. New Shakspere Soc. ed., 1878
Hawker, Footprints of Former Men in Far Cornwall, 1870
Hecker, Epidemics of the Middle Ages
Henderson, Wm. Folk-Lore of the Northern Counties, 1879
Heucherus et Fabricius. De Vegetabilibus Magicis, Wittenberg. 1700
Hunt, Robert, Popular Romances of West of England, first and second series, 1865

Irish Popular and Medical Superstitious

Jones, W., Finger Ring Lore

Keary, C. F., Outlines of Primitive Belief, 1882
Keightley, Thomas, Fairy Mythology, 1860
Kelly, W. K., Curiosities of Indo-European Traditions and Folk-Lore, 1863

Lecky, History of England in the Eighteenth Century, vol. i. ii.
Lenormant, La Magie chez les Chaldéens
Livingstone, D., South Africa
Lubbock, Sir John, The Origin of Civilization and the Primitive Condition of Man, 4th ed. 1882

Martius, Dissertatio De Magia Naturali, &c., Erfurt, 1700
Mead, Influence of Sun and Moon on Human Bodies

Mitchell, Arthur, The Past in the Present, 1880

Napier, James, Folk-Lore or Superstitious Beliefs in the West of Scotland, 1879
Nork,F., Mythologie und Volksmärchen, 1848
Notes and Queries

Pazig, De Incantationibus Magicis, 1721
Pettigrew, Superstitions connected with the Practice of Medicine and Surgery
Pratt, Anne, Wild Flowers

Ramesay, Wm., 'Ελμινθολογια, 1668
Records of the Past, vols. i. iii.

Scott, Sir W., Demonology and Witchcraft
Seton, St. Kilda Past and Present, 1878
Shakespeare Jest Books, A. C. Mery Talys, &c. 3 vols. 1864
Sinistrari, Le R. P., De la Démonialité, traduit, du Latin, par Isidore Liseux, 1879
Spalding, T. A., Elizabethan Demonology, 1880
Spencer, Herbert, Principles of Sociology, 1877
——— Study of Sociology, 1878
Stallybrass, James S., Teutonic Mythology (translation of Grimm's Deutsche Mythologie), vol. i. 1880, ii. 1883
Story, W. W., Castle of St. Angelo and the Evil Eye, 1877
Sykes, Wirt, British Goblins

Tylor, E. B., Primitive Culture, 2 vols. 1871
——— Early History of Mankind

University Magazine, August 1879, " Fairy Superstitions in Donegal "
Witches of Renfrewshire, a History of the, New Edition with Introduction, 1877

INDEX.

Abgar's letter, king, 87
Ablution, 88
Adders, bite of, 122, 123, 192
Agate, 176
Ague, cause of, 27, 95
—·— cures for, 35, 38, 39, 56, 57, 58, 59, 60, 81, 82, 86, 100, 122, 124, 152, 165, 170, 183, 192, 195, 201, 202
Alder, 57
Amaranth, 108, 201
Ancestor worship, 205
Animal Cures, Ch. x. 148
—— disease transferred to, 44
—— diseases of, transferred, 47
Ants' eggs, 193
Apple, tree and fruit, 38, 42, 57, 201
Arrow-heads, flint, 182
Ash tree, 38, 67, 195, 197, 198
—— sap, 179, 196
Ashes, 42, 72
Aspen leaf, 203
Ass, 122, 153, 158
Association of Ideas. Sympathy and, Ch. III. 49
Asthma, 125, 189

"Baaras," 195
Bats, 164
Bay tree, 154, 197 *
Bean, 57, 199
Bear, 159, 160
Beetle, 61
Bells, 19
Birth hour, 124, 128, 132
Black (colour), 115, 219
—— thorn, 57, 202
Blackberry 202
Bleeding, to stop, 76, 79, 80, 97, 111, 139, 176, 198
Blindness, 92, 185
Blood bread, 100
Bloodstone, 176
Blue, colour, 112
Boils, 42, 194
Borgie well, 103
Bramble, 70, 119

Briar rose, 199
Broom, 203
Burial, 29, 101
Burns, to cure, 80, 81, 189

Cabbage, 192, 193 *
Cake, children passed through, 69
Cancer, cause of, 31
—— to cure, 148
Cat, 44, 69, 116, 117, 151, 164
Caterpillar, 61
Cattle diseases, 55, 57, 63, 69, 74, 83, 104, 106, 112
Chader Well, 102
Charmers, 14
Cherry tree, 68
Chestnut, 193
Chilblains, 202, 203
Child-birth, 84, 90‡, 93, 100, 128, 155, 178, 182
Churchyards, 95, 96
Club moss, 76
Coal as an amulet, 219
Cock, 46, 72, 112
Cockroach, 161
Coffin handles, 175
Colic, 154, 183
Colour, Ch. VII. 108
Confirmation, 89, 187
Consumption, cause of, 26, 96
———— cures for, 31, 56, 73, 100, 161
Convulsions, cure for, 41, 86, 87, 94, 148, 189, 195
Coral, red, 22, 37
Corns, to cure, 193
Couvade, 178, 179
Cow, 69, 74, 96, 161
Crab, 161
Cramp, cause of, 27, 95
—— to cure, 86, 154, 156, 175, 182, 199
Crocodile, charm against, 50
" Crooke," the, 157
Cross, invoked, 83 ; sign of, 85, 128
—— buns, 86, 133

Crowsfoot, 201
Cuckoo, 164, 188

Dandelion, 199
Days of birth, 132
Days, holy, 133, 134, 135
Dead, cause disease, 25, 205
—— forcing disease on the, 42, 101
—— touch of, 100
"Dead men's pinches," 27
Deafness, to cure, 117, 161, 193
Death or the Grave, Charms connected with, Ch. VI. 95.
Death, theories as to cause of, 3, 4, 183, 205.
Devil, causes diseases, 10, 13, 19
—— to appease, 117
—— to invoke, 117, 170
—— charm against, 197
Devil's mark, 113, 155
Diarrhœa, to cure, 165
Digby, Sir Kenelm, on sympathy, 52
Disease, cause of, 4, 14, 25, 30, 205
—— personified, 5, 7, 8
—— burial of, 55
Disease, Transference of, Ch. II. 34
Docken, 194
Dog, 35, 117, 148
—— to cure bite of, 50, 51, 134, 196, 200, 201. *See* Hydrophobia.
—— howling of, 190
Domestic Folk-Medicine, Ch. XII. 178
Dow Loch, 103
Dreams, 129
Dropsy, to cure, 63, 174, 203
Drowning, charm against, 84
—— men, aversion to saving, 28
Dumbness, to cure, 203

Earache, to cure, 158, 160
Eel's blood, 162
Eel-skin, 161
Elder, 185, 192
Elf shots, 112
Elk's hoof, 160*
Enemy causes disease, 4, 14
Epilepsy, cause of, 126
—— to cure 46, 72, 96, 116, 120, 124, 126, 153, 162, 188, 195, 196, 202
Erysipelas, to cure, 106, 116, 139, 140, 189, 192
"Esëre," 199
Evil Eye, 21, 112, 166, 184, 201, 218
Eyebright, 200
"Faire Claidth," 29
Fairies, 165
"Feargartha," 30

Fern, 202, 203
Fever, cause of, 126
—— to cure, 35, 38, 58, 59, 62, 68, 90‡, 111, 113, 114, 119, 148, 170, 173, 174, 192, 202
Finger nails, 41, 56, 72, 181
Finger ring, 176
Fire, 69
Fir-tree, 38
Fish, transference of disease to, 36
Fits, to cure, 12, 84, 89, 95, 97, 99
Flagellation, 99, 177, 202
Flax, 185
Folk-Medicine: Origin of Disease, 1; Transference of Disease, 34; Sympathy and Association of Ideas, 49; New Berth and Sacrifice, 65; Our Lord and the Saints in, 75; Charms connected with Death and the Grave, 95; Colour, 108; Number, 118; Influence of Sun and Moon, 124; Personal Cures, 136; Animal Cures, 148; Magic Writings, 165; Rings, 172; Domestic, 178; Place of—in study of Civilization, 204
Fox, 158
Freckles, 119, 199
Frog, 35, 63, 187
Fuller's tenzle, 202
Fumitory, 201

Gallows, chips of, 100
Goat, brain, blood, horn and skin of, 162
Goitre, to cure, 101
Gold ring, 173
Good Friday Charms, 86, 133, 137
Gout, to cure, 38, 63, 90‡, 131, 164, 176, 184, 187, 189
"Grammar-sows," 198
Grass in St. Edrin's churchyard, 96
Grave, earth from, 27‡, 95
Green (colour), 114
Groundsel, 192

Hair, human, 16, 27, 72, 95, 185
Halter, 100
Hare, 31, 154
Harelip, cause of, 31, 155
Hazel, 122, 193
Headache, cause of, 11
—— to cure, 93, 96, 100, 156, 174
Hedge-hog, eye of, 186
Hellebore, 187
Hen, 116, 117, 158
Herring, 182
Hiccough, to cure, 85

INDEX.

Hoarseness, to cure, 193
Holly, 202
Horse, 117, 152
—— shoe, 154
Hydrophobia, to cure, 50, 69, 96, 120, 144, 149, 154, 167

Images, made to cause disease, 19
—— to cure disease, 64
Inflammation, to cure, 105, 115, 119
Iris, yellow, 203
Ivy, 202

Jasper, 111, 154
Jaundice, to cure, 56, 60, 115, 148, 157, 159
Juniper, 202

Keogh family, blood of, 140
King Charles I., blood of, 100
King's Evil, to cure, 62, 100, 101, 140
Kings, touch of, 140
Knife, murderer's 97
Knots, 79, 120, 185

Lark, 164
Laurel, 154, 197*, 202
Leek, juice of, 203
Left and right, 186
Leg, to cure inflammation of, 158
Leprosy, to cure, 74, 100, 156
Life absorbed in instrument of death, 99
Lightning, 11‡
—— charm against, 197*
Linnet, 164
Liver complaint, to cure, 108, 135
Lizard, 162
Loadstone, 182
Lumbago, 137
Lunacy, cause of, 6, 135
—— to cure, 45, 73, 86, 91, 102, 110, 195, 202

"Macdonald's disease," 138
Mad stone, 144
Magic Writings, Ch. XI. (1), 165
Maple, 68
Marjoram, 198
Marriage name, 138
Mary Queen of Scots' body, 28
Measles, cure for, 157, 199
Mèn-an-tol, 66
Mice, fried, 159
Midsummer Day, 135

"Milner's thumbs," 147
Mistletoe, 173, 195, 196
Mole, on right temple, 187
—— paw of, 161
Moon, Influence of the Sun and, Ch. VIII. (2), 124, 151
Moss, from skull, 96
Mouth, to cure sore, 122
Mugwort, 194, 201
Mulberry, 189
Mumps, cure for, 105

Nahak burners, 17
Names, importance of, 20, 58, 90, 138
Neck, to cure swollen, 95, 119, 156
Nettle rush, 199
Nettles, 194, 195
New Birth and Sacrifice, Ch. IV. 65
Nine (number), 57, 68, 69, 73, 79, 118
Noise, as a healer, 18
Nose-bleeding, to cure, 62, 64, 76, 97, 111, 167, 183, 191, 202
Number, Ch. VIII. (1), 118

Oak tree, 37, 39, 68
Onions, juice of, 193
Ophthalmic complaints, to cure. 63, 76, 119, 139, 144, 151, 157, 158, 161, 163, 170, 173, 191, 192, 200, 201, 202, 203
Our Lord and the Saints in Folk-Medicine, Ch. V. 75
Owl broth, eggs, &c. 164
Ox, 159

Palsy, to cure, 156
Paralysis, cause of, 14, 17, 159
—— to cure, 12, 159, 174
Peach, leaves of, 199
Pear-tree, 96
Peas, 199
Peony, 195
Personal Cures, Ch. IX. 136
Pig, bite of, 31
Pigeons, 163
Plant charms, 191
Pleurisy, to cure, 162, 163
Poison, 92, 183, 193
Potato, 182, 193
Psalms, 89, 91, 122

Queens, touch of, 143
Quinsy, to cure, 192

Radish, 203

Rainbow causes disease, 11
Rash, cause of, 27
—— to cure, 159
Red (colour), 108, 158
—— thread, 113, 197
Regeneration, 65. *See New Birth*
Rheumatism, to cure, 63, 70, 99, 152, 154, 156, 174, 177, 182, 193, 201, 202
Rickets, to cure, 56, 125
Rings, 128, 153, 172
—— cramp, 175
—— Sacrament, 174
Ringworm, to cure, 42, 123, 139, 182, 184
"Robin Redbreast's cushion," 199
Rocks, perforated, 63
Rowan, 39, 197
Rue, 200
Ruptures, to cure, 67

Sacrament rings, 174
Sacrifice, New Birth and, Ch. IV. 65
St. Apollonia, 93
— Blaze, 92
— Convall's Chariot, 104
— Edrin's churchyard, 96
— George, 93
— Guthlac's belt, 93
— John (Baptist), 91
———- Gospel, 91, 154, 167
———- Well, Wembdon, 102
— Marchutus, 94
— Nacaise, 92
— Nun's Well 102
— Peter, 77, 92
— Thomas Becket, 93
— Veronica, 94
— Victricius, 94
— Anthony's fire, to cure, 38, 190
— Vitus dance, to cure, 170, 183
Salt, 131
Scalds, to cure, 81*, 193
Scarlet fever, to cure, 35
Sciatica, to cure, 107, 203*
Scorpions, charms against, 93
Scrofula, to cure, 66, 124, 198
Seven (number), 92, 121, 129, 132
Seventh son, 122, 133, 136
—— daughters, 137
Sheep, 117, 156, 157
Shingles, cause of, 10
—————— to cure, 116, 117*, 151
Silverweed, 119, 199
Sleeping foot, to cure, 85
Sleeplessness, to cure, 154, 162, 187
Smallpox, cause of, 5, 7
—————— to cure, 7, 93, 103
Snails, 56, 157

Snakes and snake bites, 10, 45, 51, 58, 155, 158, 162, 196, 200
Sores, to cure, 75, 196
Special healers, 14, 104, 122, 133, 136, 137, 162
Specific Charms, Ch. XI. 165
Spider, 58, 59
Spine disease, to cure, 66 165
Spittle, 16, 184
Sprains, to cure, 78, 137, 161
Stag, 159
Stars, influence of, 129
Stings, to cure, 120
Stitch, to cure, 80
Stones, special powers in, 4, 7, 104, 110, 120, 144, 154
—————— transmission through, 66
Stork, eggs of, 164
"Strangers' cold," 24
Straw, 57
—— rope, 69
Suicide, touch of hand of, 101
—— ghost of, 110
Sun and Moon, Influence of, Ch. VIII. (2), 124
Sunday, 133
Swellings, to cure, 95, 113, 119, 161
Symbolic injury, 19
Sympathy and Association of Ideas, Ch. III. 49
Sympathy with natural objects, human, 31, 67

Taoist priests, 21
Tetter, to cure, 123. *See* Ringworm
Thorn, to cure prick, 82, 83
Throat, to cure sore, 106, 116, 182, 192
Thrush, to cure, 35, 104, 138
Thunder, charm against, 197 †
Thyme, 198
Tigretier, to cure, 92
Toad, 17, 31, 42, 58, 62, 63
Toad doctor, 61
Tooth from corpse, 98
Toothache, cause of, 11, 32
—————— to cure, 14, 33, 35, 38, 63, 77, 89, 90*, 93, 98, 119, 139, 156, 161, 171, 177, 182, 187, 188, 192, 193, 196, 202, 203
Transference of Disease, Ch. II. 34
Trees, 37, 39, 67, 73
—— transmission through, 31, 67
Tripe, 200
Twin, a "left," 138

Ulcerations, to cure, 100, 139
Unbaptized children, 98

Vervain, 135, 153, 193
Vulture's leg and toes, sinews of, 164

Warts, cause of, 30, 31, 187
—— to cure, 38, 41, 43, 56, 86, 126, 127, 130, 138, 151, 152. 158, 162, 168, 173, 185, 192, 199
Watercresses, 192
Waterlilies, 12
Water-spirits, 12, 28, 116
Waters, Holy, 31, 39, 40, 46, 73. 88, 89, 92, 102, 103, 104, 133, 179
Weakness, to cure, 201
Wedding-ring, 173
Wells, See Waters, Holy, supra
Wens, to cure, 168. See Warts

White (colour), 115
Whooping-cough, to cure, 35, 36, 61, 70, 88, 89, 90, 101, 106, 111, 118, 119, 120, 138, 153, 157, 159, 182, 183, 199

"Widderschynnes," 130, 131
Willow, 38, 58
Wisewomen, See Special Healers and Witchcraft
Witchcraft, witches, wizards, &c., 9, 10, 12, 14, 15, 19, 26, 69, 83, 89, 96, 185, 188, 192, 197†, 199, 203
Wolf, 92, 153. 154
Woodbine, 68
Worms, to cure, 199
Wounds, to heal, 76, 79, 148, 193, 198, 199, 202

Yarrow, 201
Yellow (colour), 108, 115

ERRATA.

163. *For* " in January, five years, later Kate Joyce," &c., *read* " in January, five years later, Kate Joyce," &c.

169. *For* " the little figure of the sick man," &c., *read* " the little finger of the sick man," &c.

194. *For* " Glasgow," *read* " Port Glasgow."

199. *For* " the excrescence found on a briar sore," *read* " the excrescence found on a briar rose."

www.ingramcontent.com/pod-product-compliance
Lightning Source LLC
Chambersburg PA
CBHW031750230426
43669CB00007B/565